The ABCs of CBM

A Practical Guide to Curriculum-Based Measurement

MICHELLE K. HOSP
JOHN L. HOSP
KENNETH W. HOWELL

THE GUILFORD PRESS
New York   London

Library of Congress Cataloging-in-Publication Data

Hosp, Michelle K.
    The ABCs of CBM : a practical guide to curriculum-based measurement / Michelle K. Hosp, John L. Hosp, Kenneth W. Howell.
        p. cm. — (The Guilford practical intervention in the schools series)
    ISBN-10: 1-59385-399-8   ISBN-13: 978-1-59385-399-0 (pbk.: alk. paper)
    1. Curriculum-based assessment—United States.   2. Educational tests and measurements—United States.   I. Hosp, John L.   II. Howell, Kenneth W.   III. Title.
    LB3060.32.C74H67 2006
    371.2′64—dc22
                                                                    2006027886

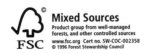
Mixed Sources
Product group from well-managed
forests, and other controlled sources
www.fsc.org Cert no. SW-COC-002358
FSC   © 1996 Forest Stewardship Council

About the Authors

Michelle K. Hosp, PhD, is a Research Associate in the Department of Special Education at the University of Utah. She earned her doctorate in education and human development from the Peabody College of Education at Vanderbilt University and her master's in school psychology from the Rochester Institute of Technology. Her research focus is on using curriculum-based measurement (CBM) to inform instruction in the area of reading. Dr. Hosp has been using CBM and conducting trainings for more than 10 years and is also a trainer for the National Center on Student Progress Monitoring.

John L. Hosp, PhD, is an Assistant Professor in the School of Teacher Education at Florida State University and Research Faculty at the Florida Center for Reading Research. He has a master's degree in school psychology from the Rochester Institute of Technology and a doctorate in education and human development from the Peabody College of Education at Vanderbilt University. His research interests include disproportionate representation of minority students in special education, aligning assessment with intervention, and the design and implementation of response to intervention (RTI). Dr. Hosp has used CBM extensively in his own practice as a school psychologist and has trained educators in several states to use CBM and DIBELS.

Kenneth W. Howell, PhD, is a Professor in the Department of Special Education at Western Washington University. Dr. Howell has published extensively in the areas of curriculum-based evaluation (CBE), CBM, and evaluation. His primary areas of research interest are problem solving, RTI, CBE, CBM, and school violence. A former special education teacher and school psychologist, Dr. Howell is well known in both fields as a speaker and trainer.

Contents

1. **What Is CBM and Why Should I Do It?** 1

   What Will I Learn from This Book? 2

   What Is CBM? 2

   Why Were the Other Attributes, Like the Timing and Charting, Developed? 3

   How Is CBM Different from Other Forms of Measurement? 5

   Curriculum 5

   Alterable Variables 6

   Low-Inference Measures 6

   Criterion-Referenced Measures 7

   What Are the Main Advantages of CBM? 8

   What Kind of Decisions Can I Make with CBM Data? 9

   How Does CBM Relate to RTI? 9

   So CBM Does Just About Everything? 10

   Are There Different Types of CBM? 10

   General Outcome Measures 10

   Skills-Based Measures 11

   Mastery Measures 12

   I Have Never Seen CBM Being Used. If It's So Great, Why Isn't It More Popular? 14

   Is CBM Used in Special Education or General Education? 16

   Who Gives CBM Measures? 16

   If I Want to Use CBM, Does This Mean I'll Need to Make Tests Out of the Instructional Materials I'm Using? 17

   Where Do I Get CBM Materials? 18

2. **CBM for Assessment and Problem Solving** 19

   What Do I Need to Know about Educational Decision Making? 20

   What Is a Criterion-Referenced Test? 22

   Are CBMs Standardized Tests? 24

   How Reliable and Valid Is CBM? 24

   Where Do They Get the Performance Standards Used in CBM? 25

   How Can CBM Be Used for Screening/Benchmarking? 26

   Screening Summary 27

   How Can CBM Be Used for Progress Monitoring? 27

   Progress Monitoring Summary 28

   So Where Do We Go from Here? 29

3. How to Conduct Reading CBM   31

   Overview of Why to Conduct Reading CBM   31
   ORF CBM   32
      Materials Needed to Conduct ORF CBM   32
      Directions and Scoring Procedures for ORF CBM   35
   Maze CBM   40
      Materials Needed to Conduct Maze CBM   40
      Directions and Scoring Procedures for Maze CBM   42
   How Often Should ORF and Maze CBM Be Given?   44
   How Much Time Does It Take to Administer and Score Reading CBM?   46
   Expected Growth Rates and Norms for ORF and Maze CBM   46
      How Much Progress Can We Expect in Reading?   46
      Proficiency Levels or Benchmarks for Reading CBM   48
      Norms for Reading CBM   48
   Survey-Level Assessment with ORF CBM   51
   How to Use the Information to Write Reading IEP Goals and Objectives   51
   Frequently Asked Questions about Reading CBM   53

4. How to Conduct Early Reading CBM   55

   Overview of Why to Conduct Early Reading CBM   55
   Overview of DIBELS Measures   56
      Initial Sound Fluency and Phoneme Segmentation Fluency   56
      Nonsense Word Fluency   57
      Letter Naming Fluency   57
   LSF CBM   57
      Materials Needed to Conduct LSF CBM   57
      Directions and Scoring Procedures for LSF CBM   59
   WIF CBM   63
      Materials Needed to Conduct WIF CBM   63
      Directions and Scoring Procedure for WIF CBM   64
   How Often Should LSF and WIF CBM Be Given?   67
   How Much Time Does It Take to Administer and Score Early Reading CBM?   68
   Expected Growth Rates and Norms for LSF and WIF CBM   68
      Proficiency Levels or Benchmarks for Early Reading CBM   68
      Norms for Early Reading CBM   68
   How to Use the Information to Write Early Reading IEP Goals and Objectives   69
   Frequently Asked Questions about Early Reading CBM   70

5. How to Conduct Spelling CBM   72
   with TESSIE ROSE

   Overview of Why to Conduct Spelling CBM   72
   Materials Needed to Conduct Spelling CBM   72
      Spelling CBM Lists   73
   Directions and Scoring Procedures for Spelling CBM   75
      Directions for Spelling CBM   75
      Scoring Spelling CBM   76
   How Often Should Spelling CBM Be Given?   78
   How Much Time Does It Take to Administer and Score Spelling CBM?   78
   Expected Growth Rates and Norms for Spelling CBM   79
      How Much Progress Can We Expect in Spelling?   79
      Norms for Spelling CBM   80
   How to Use the Information to Write Spelling IEP Goals and Objectives   80
   Frequently Asked Questions about Spelling CBM   80

6.　How to Conduct Writing CBM　　　　84
　　with TESSIE ROSE
　　Overview of Why to Conduct Writing CBM　84
　　Materials Needed to Conduct Writing CBM　85
　　　Writing CBM Story Starters　85
　　Directions and Scoring Procedures for Writing CBM　88
　　　Directions for Writing CBM　88
　　　Scoring Writing CBM　88
　　How Often Should Writing CBM Be Given?　93
　　How Much Time Does It Take to Administer and Score Writing CBM?　93
　　Expected Growth Rates and Norms for Writing CBM　93
　　How to Use the Information to Write Writing IEP Goals and Objectives　94
　　Frequently Asked Questions about Writing CBM　94

7.　How to Conduct Math CBM　　　　97
　　Overview of Why to Conduct Math CBM　97
　　Materials Needed to Conduct Math CBM　98
　　　Math CBM Sheets　98
　　Directions and Scoring Procedures for Math CBM　104
　　　Directions for Math CBM　104
　　　Scoring Math CBM　104
　　How Often Should Math CBM Be Given?　108
　　How Much Time Does It Take to Administer and Score Math CBM?　108
　　Expected Growth Rates and Norms for Math CBM　109
　　　How Much Progress Can We Expect in Math?　109
　　　Proficiency Levels or Benchmarks for Math CBM　109
　　　Norms for Math CBM　109
　　Survey-Level Assessment with Math CBM　110
　　How to Use the Information to Write Math IEP Goals and Objectives　111
　　Special Considerations That Apply to Math CBM　112
　　　Accuracy of Teacher/Examiner Copy　112
　　　Setting Up Math CBM Sheets to Provide Potential Diagnostic Information　112
　　　Early Numeracy　113
　　　Concepts and Applications　115
　　　Estimation　115
　　Frequently Asked Questions About Math CBM　116

8.　Charting and Graphing Data to Help Make Decisions　　　　118
　　Procedures and Materials Needed to Chart CBM Data　118
　　How to Set and Graph Goals　120
　　　End-of-Year Benchmarks　120
　　　Norms　121
　　　Intraindividual Framework　122
　　　Graphing Goals　123
　　How Often Should Data Be Collected?　123
　　Decision Rules to Help Educators Use the Data to Inform Instruction　124
　　Considerations for Graphing and Charting the Data in the Content Areas　126
　　The Use of CBM in Response to Intervention　126
　　Computerized Graphing and Data Management Systems　127
　　　Material-Specific Programs　128
　　　Material-Flexible Programs　129
　　　Spreadsheet and Data Management Programs　130
　　Frequently Asked Questions about Charting and Graphing CBM Data　130

9. **Planning to Use CBM—and Keeping It Going**   132
Developing a Plan for Using CBM   132
    Ten Steps to Using CBM before, during, and after Initial Implementation   133
Hints on How to Get CBM Going   138
Hints on How to Keep CBM Going   138
Frequently Asked Questions about Planning and Using CBM   139

Appendix A. Summary of Validity and Reliability Studies for CBM   141

Appendix B. Reproducible Quick Guides and Forms for Conducting CBM   143

References   163

Index   167

The ABCs of CBM

1

What Is CBM
and Why Should I Do It?

This book is about an assessment tool called *curriculum-based measurement* (CBM). The book begins by explaining a little bit about what CBM is and where it came from, but the majority of it will focus on the nuts and bolts (i.e., the ABCs) of how to use CBM in a classroom, school, or district to improve the quality of educational decision making.

Given the number of assessment and evaluation initiatives that are loose in education today, you might be wondering why you need to know about another. That is a legitimate question, and the first thing we want to let you know is that we are not presenting CBM as something *additional* to do. CBM is an alternative to other procedures you may already be doing or that you may be avoiding because they are too time consuming or complex to justify. Every minute spent on assessing takes time away from teaching. Therefore, assessments should be efficient and provide information that will guide instruction and improve student outcomes. This is the premise behind our approach to evaluation.

Imagine that you are planning a business trip and you need to fly somewhere. You have your choice of many different airlines, fares, schedules, seating options, and routes. The last flight you took (on Traditional Air) was expensive. In addition, the schedules didn't accommodate your work day, the seats weren't made for someone your size, and the flight, because it wasn't direct, took forever. But now there is an alternative carrier: Air CBM. Air CBM goes directly where you want to go in less time for half the price! In addition, it flies when you want, and the seats are adjustable. Which option will you pick? Our guess is that you would pick Air CBM. You certainly wouldn't decide to fly both airlines and make the same trip twice for one day's work.

1

Here are the first two things you need to know about CBM:

1. CBM is not an "add on." CBM is an alternative. In some cases it is an alternative to assessments that are too costly, time consuming, or disruptive to instruction. This means that by employing CBM you may actually be able to get more done—not less.
2. CBM is a bargain. CBM gets you where you are going by helping you improve student learning in less time and with less cost.

WHAT WILL I LEARN FROM THIS BOOK?

This book will teach you a set of skills that lead to quality instruction. It is basically a book about collecting and using information. Whenever we work at something important, it is best to develop a plan before we start and to check on our progress while we are working. This allows us to work in an intentional and thoughtful way. It also gives us an idea about what we are trying to accomplish and alerts us when we need to change if what we are doing isn't getting us closer to that goal. Because educating children, adolescents, and young adults certainly fits within the definition of an important activity, it makes sense that the process of doing it should include things like goal setting, planning, and monitoring. To do these things well, an educator needs information, and the quality of the information you have will, in large part, determine the quality of the work you do.

We have all read or heard of the many reports documenting the need for improved services in certain content areas and for some particularly vulnerable groups of students. In the United States, for example, there are literally millions of school-age students (ages 6–21) with serious reading problems. Similarly, it is widely recognized that students coming from low-income families or belonging to certain linguistic or racial/ethnic groups are less likely to succeed in school. As a result, educators have an increased responsibility to make informed decisions when working to teach important skills like reading and when tackling the needs of students who face problems learning. It is difficult for teachers to think their way through these important efforts without something concrete to think about.

We believe that CBM provides exactly the kind of functional information required to inform educational decision making. The purpose of this book is to teach you how to get and use that information so that more students will succeed in school.

WHAT IS CBM?

CBM is an assessment tool characterized by certain attributes. We'll explain these attributes, but first you should know what CBM "looks" like.

CBM is usually composed of a set of standard directions, a timing device, a set of materials (i.e., passages, sheets, lists), scoring rules, standards for judging performance, and record forms or charts. The directions given are very straightforward in that they ask the student to engage in a task that is not that different than something she would usually do during class (e.g., read from a book, write a paragraph, or solve computation problems). The materials the student works on will look just like class materials. When the student performs these tasks, you'll see that she is timed so that her level of performance can be scored in terms of the number of responses correct and incorrect per minute—the person giving the test will have some sort of timer. You will also probably see the student's level of performance on the test charted on a graph or entered into a computer so that trends in her learning can be analyzed over time.

Because you won't see the performance standards or the scoring rules, if you didn't know what you were looking for you might not even recognize the administration of the CBM measures as an evaluation. It will look very much like a teaching activity. That is because one of the supporting principles of CBM is an idea called *alignment*. The principle of alignment basically holds that your educational efforts will be more effective if you "test what you teach and teach what you test." *What* you teach is called the *curriculum*. It is the goals and objectives that must be met to achieve social and academic competence. (This is a fairly standard definition. The word *curriculum* comes from the Latin word *currer* for racing chariots. The curriculum, then, is the "course" to be followed to reach the finish line.)

WHY WERE THE OTHER ATTRIBUTES, LIKE THE TIMING AND CHARTING, DEVELOPED?

CBM evolved out of work by Stan Deno and Phyllis Mirkin in the late 1970s and early 1980s at the Minnesota Institute for Research on Learning Disabilities. They were working on an intervention process called Data-Based Program Modification (DBPM). DBPM was a complete package of procedures for establishing goals, planning interventions (with a heavy emphasis on collaboration and consultation), and monitoring. In order for DBPM to work, there needed to be a continuous data collection system in place to produce the information required to guide the decisions that fueled the program modifications. It was also needed because, as many of the instructional interventions were designed through consultation, the person delivering the lessons was not always the person responsible for the students' learning.

Deno and Mirkin soon realized that they needed an assessment system built on a set of common principles and composed of standardized procedures and rules. In a way, this sort of system already existed in the form of applied behavior analysis for areas such as classroom and social behavior, but it did not exist for academic content. So Deno and Mirkin began developing CBM to fill that need.

CBM is characterized by several attributes (Deno, 2003):

1. The first and most obvious is *alignment*. With CBM the students are tested on the curriculum they are being taught. This means:

- The content is the same.
- The stimulus materials the student is given look the same; the responses she is expected to make are the same.

2. The measures are *technically adequate*, meaning that they have established reliability and validity. Even though CBM is used within classrooms by teachers, it is not informal assessment. Informal assessments typically have not been shown to be technically adequate.

CBM is an empirically supported process with substantial technical adequacy. Over the past 25 years, there have been hundreds of solid empirical research studies in excellent journals supporting the application of CBM. In fact, because CBM is used to summarize both a student's level of performance and her rate of progress, it has been examined in ways that traditional measures have never been.

3. CBM typically makes use of *criterion-referenced measures* as opposed to norm-referenced measures (we'll explain this later).

4. *Standard procedures* are used. All those using CBM who want to share their data with others (for example, as part of a program evaluation or a formal student report) follow the same administration and scoring rules:

- Standard tasks are used for each content area (e.g., three 1-minute timed oral readings are used to find a student's current level of reading performance).
- Standard procedures are followed for selecting or constructing testing materials.
- Standard administration and scoring directions exist for each procedure.

5. *Performance sampling* is used (producing what is sometimes called *behavioral* or *performance data*). CBM procedures employ direct, *low-inference* measures through which correct and incorrect student behaviors on clearly defined tasks are counted within a set time interval (usually in minutes). Therefore, inference and conjecture about the meaning of the resulting scores is kept to a minimum. For example, a reading CBM might tell you that the student read a grade-level passage at "47 words correct per minute with no errors."

6. Decision rules are put in place to provide those who use the data with information about what it means when students score at different levels of performance or illustrate different rates of progress on the measures over time. These rules are based on performance criteria and are standardized through sampling or experimental procedures.

7. CBM emphasizes *repeated measurement* over time and can be used to generate rate of progress as well as level of performance data. This means that CBM data can be used for *progress monitoring* to illustrate the rate of learning as it is occurring. This allows immediate adjustments in a student's educational program when needed.

Because CBM measures what is being taught, and learning is a change in performance over time, these repeated measures illustrate the degree to which an instructional intervention is producing learning. As a result, the combined use of CBM and progress monitoring allows educators to judge the quality of instruction and to decide when changes need to be made. Therefore, CBM data don't just help teachers decide *what* to teach, they can also help them decide *how* to teach.

8. CBM is also *efficient*. It is efficient in implementation because people can be trained to give the measures in a short period of time and the measures can be given quickly. It communicates efficiently because it produces *performance* data or *behavior* data. (All educational and psychological measures require students to engage in behavior, but in many cases the original behavior, which is usually called the *raw score*, needs to be converted into another form before it can be used.) When you use performance data, you draw conclusions directly from what the student actually did on the test. There is no need to convert the raw score for most purposes. For example, if a student reads 47 words per minute and the criterion for this passage is 60 words per minute, then the conclusion is that she is reading 13 words per minute slower than she should. For classroom purposes, the results are summarized and interpreted as simple behavioral/performance statements and need not be converted into percentiles or normal-curve equivalents to be understood. All you need to know is that the student should read 13 words per minute faster than her current rate.

9. Finally, depending on need, the CBM data can be *summarized efficiently* by using a variety of techniques ranging from pencil and paper charts to web-based data management systems. This efficiency makes the data immediately accessible to any level of the educational system. Most important, it makes the data accessible to classroom teachers and students.

HOW IS CBM DIFFERENT FROM OTHER FORMS OF MEASUREMENT?

Many of the most important differences are spelled out in the nine attributes listed above, but there are some more fundamental ideas that support those attributes.

Anyone who has spent time around education knows that there are all kinds of assessments available in schools. These range in structure from statewide accountability tests to simple handwriting rubrics. In education, we use these measures to collect information in order to inform our decision making, and the form these measures take usually has a lot to do with the function they are designed to fulfill. Because there are different kinds of decisions to make and different ways to go about making these decisions, there are different forms of measures. CBM, as explained above, was designed to help teachers plan instruction and monitor it to see if it is working. There are four ways the structure of CBM reflects this instructional orientation: (1) by focusing on the curriculum; (2) by using alterable variables; (3) by employing low-inference measures; and (4) by employing criterion-referenced measures.

Curriculum

When we say a measure is curriculum-based, we are saying that it is tied to the curriculum and that, as a result, we expect to see that measure doing a good job of sampling things that students are taught. This might not be the case for measures based on ideas about general achievement, disability type, learning style, fixed ability (e.g., intelligence or cognitive ability), developmental stages, or perceptual processing. These tests may not be built to target the content a student is being taught. In fact, they may have been written to avoid it.

You probably were not surprised by the last paragraph. Our guess is that you would have anticipated that curriculum-based measures would reflect the curriculum. But CBM was also designed to function within a problem-solving paradigm or system based on systematic instructional intervention and student mastery of performance goals (e.g., response to intervention [RTI]). That system needs direct measurement of student learning to function. Measures designed to function in other problem-solving paradigms, such as the traditional student-deficit model or those that assume that instruction should yield a normal distribution of skills, are designed differently. So how are they different?

Alterable Variables

One of the most important differences between CBM and other measures used in education is that CBM targets alterable variables. In education, an *alterable variable* is something that can be changed through instruction. Performance on curricular tasks is considered alterable because it is under the direct control of teachers (i.e., it can be changed through instruction). CBM was not designed simply to document the existence of problems or to determine their cause. It was designed to fill the need for a data collection system that would produce the information required to guide instruction. One of the things CBM can do very well, for example, is tell a teacher about a student's knowledge of a particular skill. This information has immediate implications for instruction because knowledge of skills can be changed through instruction (because instruction, by definition, is the provision of new knowledge).

There is considerable debate about whether measures of unalterable student-centered variables like perceptual processing, developmental stage, or learning style provide information that is useful for guiding instruction. More to the point, the status of a student's curricular skills can be changed by the teacher through instruction, whereas things like learning style, cognitive ability, and even general achievement are conceptualized as being relatively stable. Time spent measuring them, assuming the measures work, is time spent looking at something that teachers can't do anything about. (Even if measures of those variables do work, the information they yield will still be useless without good information about what skills a student needs to learn—so, in the end, CBM is always needed.)

Low-Inference Measures

Tools that measure one thing so that conclusions can be drawn about something else require us to make *inferences*. Those that require us to measure one thing and then process the results by way of some theoretical application are called *high-inference* measures. For example, a cognitive ability test does not have any cognitive ability items on it, but it does have items from which the test user is expected to make inferences about the student's cognitive ability. Therefore, while a student may assemble geometric shapes out of blocks on a cognitive ability test, the score is not reported in terms of geometric shape production, but in terms of cognitive ability. We can only accept that interpretation of the test behavior if we accept the theory of cognitive ability on which the inference is based.

The fact that CBM is designed to sample the observable student behaviors that occur in a classroom distinguishes it from the high-inference measures often used in education and school psychology. CBM was not developed to explain how learning does or doesn't occur, and it was not designed to conform to any particular theory about how students think, attend, remember, or process information. Therefore, inference and conjecture about what the resulting scores mean is kept to a minimum. Curriculum-based measures employ direct (low-inference) observations during which correct and incorrect student responses to real tasks are counted within a set time interval (usually in minutes). If the student works seven addition fact problems in 1 minute, her score is reported as "seven addition facts per minute." If the criterion for addition facts is 40 per minute, the implication of the seven-per-minute score is simple: The student needs instruction on addition.

Criterion-Referenced Measures

Another way that CBM is different from most traditional educational and psychological measures is that it escapes the normative tradition and employs criterion-referenced measures (although norms for many of the measures are also available). Criterion-referenced measures are used to determine if students can demonstrate their knowledge by reaching specified performance levels (i.e., criteria) on certain tasks. The basic assumption is that students who do not know a skill and need instruction on it will do poorly on the test of that skill. Those who *do* know the skill will pass the test.

One of the biggest problems with the utility of educational evaluation is that its history has been grounded almost exclusively in normative comparison and the use of normative measures. There is nothing wrong with normative comparison or the measures used to conduct it as long as your goal is to find out how a student's level of performance compares to the level of performance of others, but that usually isn't the most important thing teachers need to know. For planning a lesson, it is more important to know if the student has or hasn't mastered the skills about to be covered or how she should best be taught the things she doesn't know. Knowing how a student compares to other students does not provide that information.

CBM came directly out of an intervention program and was designed to inform teachers' decisions about *what* and *how* to teach. As has already been explained, it was designed to provide measures with instructional utility. This meant that the measures had to be:

- Aligned with curriculum;
- Sensitive to instruction;

- Repeatable so that progress monitoring could occur; and
- Criterion-referenced so that they could be used to determine when a student had mastered a task.

This allows teachers to set goals, determine the level of a student's prerequisite knowledge, align instruction with outcomes, and track progress toward goals.

WHAT ARE THE MAIN ADVANTAGES OF CBM?

If we have to pick a few advantages, we will go with efficiency, alignment, and usefulness in progress monitoring. The first one, efficiency, is important because no one is going to use a measure that is awkward, confusing, or burdensome. CBM is actually quite simple to use and to understand. This means less time assessing and more time teaching.

The second choice would have to be CBM's *alignment*, or linkage, with instructional outcomes. Alignment between measurement and the curriculum being taught allows the user to make better decisions. For example, alignment improves decisions about what the student can and can't do. As you will see, CBM lets us be very precise when selecting instructional goals and determining current levels of performance. Alignment is often lost in traditional normative measures constructed by using a sample of items selected across a wide range of difficulty. (You're familiar with this format. It is the one that starts with very easy items and moves quickly through increasingly complex material.) In order to cover a range of skills and keep such tests down to a manageable size, the curricular distance between the items on these tests is often large, and very few items are provided for each skill. Alignment is lost because of the limited sampling (i.e., the number of items for each skill) and because some skills are completely left off the test.

Alignment is also lost when measures use item formats that present the student with tasks different from those he actually needs to use. For example, group-administered tests often ask students to identify answers by circling or matching them. In actual practice, students don't usually identify the correct answers; they produce them. These are two different skills.

Our third choice is CBM's usefulness for progress monitoring. Typical normative achievement measures can't be used to decide if instruction is working within a fairly short period of time because they are designed to yield scores that are highly stable over time (a student's score on the test isn't meant to change across short periods) and they don't have a sufficient number of alternate forms for frequent retesting. CBM allows for progress monitoring by using equivalent samples in a repeated (even daily) measurement format. Frequent use coupled with alignment makes CBM more sensitive to instruction than typical measures. This means it can be used to decide, within a fairly short period of time, when instruction is (or isn't) working and that means CBM can also be used to help one decide *how* to teach. It does this by letting us see, in a timely manner, when instruction is working and when it should be changed.

By opening up access to progress data, CBM supplies educators with a whole new assembly of information that can be used to make a whole new set of informed decisions. The use of information collected during the process of instruction is called *formative evaluation*. Formative evaluation was a central component of the DBPM system originally developed by Deno and Mirkin. It involves the use of information from repeated direct measures to display trends in learning so that instructional decisions can be made based on levels of student progress. This is, hands down, the most powerful tool available to a teacher or school psychologist!

WHAT KIND OF DECISIONS CAN I MAKE WITH CBM DATA?

As will be explained in Chapter 2, there are four major kinds of decisions we make in education:

1. *Screening decisions* to decide which students need help and which don't;
2. *Progress-monitoring decisions* to decide when to move on to new goals or modify instruction;
3. *Diagnostic decisions* to decide what kind of help a student needs; and
4. *Outcome decisions* to decide when special services can be discontinued and to document the overall effectiveness of efforts across all students.

While CBM data can be used to inform each of these types of decisions, the kinds of measures we use and the way we use them depend on which of these decisions we are trying to make. For example, during the screening and diagnostic functions, we may do something called *survey-level assessment*. Survey-level assessments collect a broad sample of the student's behavior in a content area in order to:

1. Find the student's instructional level; and
2. Check quickly the student's level of performance in order to narrow the scope of additional testing.

When survey-level assessment indicates a problem, someone doing a diagnostic evaluation may follow it with *specific-level* assessment to determine what and how the student needs to be taught. As will be explained shortly, *general outcome* and *skills-based* CBMs are often used as survey measures and *mastery measure* CBMs are often used as specific measures.

HOW DOES CBM RELATE TO RTI?

RTI often means different things to different people, but in general it includes the use of data-based decision making for various problem-solving tasks. Key components of any good RTI approach are the use of screening/benchmarking and progress-monitoring assessments. As mentioned above (and in more depth in Chapter 2), CBM is an excellent way to approach making both of these types of decisions. In Chapter 8 we elaborate on how CBM fits into RTI.

SO CBM DOES JUST ABOUT EVERYTHING?

Well, it doesn't teach!

CBM is *not* an instructional method or intervention. It is a tool for improving instruction that is compatible with diverse instructional approaches. Similarly, CBM is *not* a curriculum. So there isn't a CBM reading program.

CBM is a measurement overlay, which means the CBM administration and scoring rules are like templates that can be laid over goals and objectives from an assortment of content areas. This makes CBM uniquely valuable in situations where different teachers may be using different instructional methods or the same teacher may have different students being taught in different ways.

There are sets of published CBM measures that have been developed around particular sequences of goals, but the tasks and goal sequences used in those measures are not the defining elements of CBM (they are defining elements of the different tasks and curriculums on which they are based). The defining elements of CBM are the curriculum-based procedures for designing, administering, and scoring measures and for recording, summarizing, and interpreting the data that result from those measures. Therefore, you can't buy one CBM that will be useful for all subject areas or in all classrooms (at least not until all educators decide that they are going to teach the same things in the same sequence).

ARE THERE DIFFERENT TYPES OF CBM?

A measure gets to be a CBM instrument if it is designed, administered, and scored according to established CBM procedures. Three types of CBM procedures have been described: general outcome measures, skills-based measures, and mastery measures. These all share the eight qualities listed above but differ in design according to their purposes and the nature of the skills they are designed to test.

General Outcome Measures

General outcome measures (GOMs) are used to sample performance across several goals at the same time by using capstone tasks that are complex in the sense that they can only be accomplished by successfully applying a number of contributing skills. In this measurement format, the contributing skills (i.e., subskills) are not separated out for direct attention as they are in the skills-based measures and mastery measures we'll describe shortly. Instead, success or improvement on the GOM is assumed to reflect the synthetic application of the contributing skills. In this sense, GOMs are holistic, while mastery measures, in particular, are atomistic.

Probably the best common example of a GOM is oral reading fluency. In order for a student to read fluently (i.e., accurately and quickly), she must be able to use a variety of skills at the same time, including the skills to use letters, letter combinations, blending, vocabulary, syntax, and content knowledge. As a student improves in any of these skills, you can expect to see some improvement in her oral reading fluency. As a result, using oral reading as the GOM relieves you of the need to test each of these subskills separately (whether they are taught in isolation or in combination).

There are several obvious advantages to GOMs. The first is that they dramatically cut down on the number of different measures one has to develop, introduce, manage, administer, score, and track. By developing four or five GOMs to cover the areas addressed throughout a year, a teacher can have her monitoring system for the whole year in place on the first day. The use of GOMs also recognizes the limitations of isolating subskills from the context in which they normally are expected to function. Any time you present tasks in a format that is different from the way they will usually be used (for example, asking students to read nonsense words or the sounds of letters in isolation), there is the risk that you will lose validity. A final advantage is that visual displays of progress on a GOM will show longer acquisition slopes, allowing adequate opportunities for progress monitoring and data-based instructional modifications.

For the reasons listed above, GOMs are especially useful for screening, progress monitoring, and collecting a general sample during survey-level testing to get an overview of level of performance. The primary disadvantage of GOMs is the downside of all general procedures: they are *general.* If your student's oral reading is inadequate and you think you need specific information about her relative skill patterns, you may not get that information from a GOM. Another limitation of GOMs is that some curriculum areas do not have a capstone task that represents the synthetic application of most of the content (especially one that is reasonably convenient to use). For example, GOMs are difficult to develop in mathematics beyond the early grades.

Skills-Based Measures

Skills-based measures (SBMs) are designed to accomplish many of the functions of GOMs. They also have their particular advantages and disadvantages. Their main advantages are that they can be used to screen, progress monitor, and do survey-level assessment in curriculum domains where capstone tasks are not available.

The best example of a SBM is probably math computation. At any particular grade level, a math curriculum for computation is made up of a list of specific skills. For example, a second-grade curriculum might include addition facts, double-digit addition without regrouping, double-digit addition with regrouping, and subtraction facts. There is no single task to demonstrate proficiency on all of these skills—each needs to be measured directly, using an SBM.

SBMs are constructed by first identifying the set of goals that will be taught within a curriculum area. The time frame you will cover could sample goals for an entire year or for shorter periods. Once the goals have been identified, items are then prepared to assess each goal. The items for the same goal should be of equal difficulty. Next, the items are placed in random order (from the student's perspective) into a set of tests. This produces a set of equivalent measures providing balanced coverage of the same content.

The items on these tests are not placed in the order in which they are taught or in order of complexity. All of the items covering the same goal are not grouped together. Items should be arranged so that each goal is equally represented in each section (i.e., beginning, middle, and end) of the test. It is good to note what skills each item is measuring, however, so that you can link performance on the measure back to instructional objectives.

SBMs are generally administered by including directions like "Work as many items as you can. If you come to one you don't know, you can skip it." When given these directions and measures constructed as we have described them, students who are beginning to work on a set of skills will skip many problems and get lower scores. As they progress through the curriculum and learn new skills, their scores will improve because there will be more items they can work. Therefore, SBMs can sometimes be used to progress monitor, as they will produce long acquisition slopes like GOMs do. In addition, they can yield some analytical information as long as steps are taken to ensure that an adequate sample of each kind of item is provided and that the items are cross-referenced to goals.

One big disadvantage of SBMs is that when instruction begins, most of the items will be irrelevant to the student because they will be above her current level of performance. Near the end of instruction, most of the items will again be irrelevant because she will have already learned them. Basically, this means that at any given time only a few items on the test will be directly related to what the student is currently learning.

Mastery Measures

The last type of CBM is the mastery measure (MM). MMs differ from GOMs and SBMs in several ways, mainly in the relative levels within the curriculum from which tasks are drawn and the relative sizes of the measurement net they spread. (The term *measurement net* refers to the size and nature of the sample a measure collects. For example, a test covering 25 computation skills would be casting a larger measurement net than one covering five skills.) GOMs present tasks that are relatively more complex and/or advanced than do MMs; SBMs tend to cover more skills than MMs (i.e., they measure more by casting a wider net). Therefore, MMs are generally used on parts of the curriculum that contain discrete and easily identified sets (or domains) of items that are closely related by some common skill, theme, concept, or solution strategy. Examples of this sort of domain might include punctuation (for writing), multiplying fractions (for math), or sounds of letters (for early reading).

MMs are used in three situations:

1. When you really want to focus on a particular set of skills. These might include the so-called *tool skills*, which need to be performed at high levels of proficiency (e.g., letter formation, using the silent *e* to convert vowels, computation facts). Focus might also be important for skills that are pivotal to many other operations, like quickly going through the steps of multiplying fractions;
2. When you are trying to troubleshoot a problem and need to do specific-level testing (for example, to see if a student is having trouble with reading comprehension because he doesn't know how to tell relevant from irrelevant information); and
3. To monitor learning when a skill is being taught in isolation. (It is important to note that, even if an MM focuses on an isolated skill, it does not mean that skill should be taught in isolation. The skill is measured in isolation only for purposes of focus.)

The disadvantages of MMs come with their narrow focus. They are not good for surveying general levels of performance or for monitoring growth on long-term goals. Using a series of MMs to progress monitor will produce a profile of closely packed peaks and valleys that look like the teeth on a saw blade (see Figure 1.1). This profile emerges because, as soon as a student starts getting high scores on one of the very specific mea-

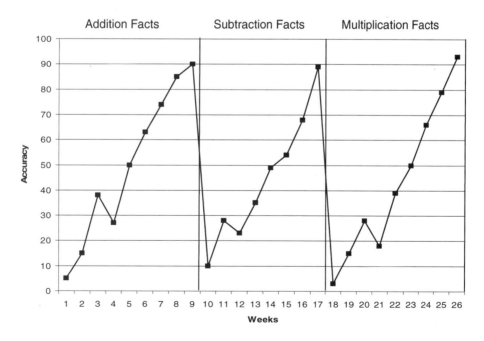

FIGURE 1.1. Example of an MM progress-monitoring profile.

sures, a new one is introduced, and her score goes back down. That is called a *measurement shift* (or as we sometimes like to call it, "jumping off cliffs"). A GOM or SBM covering what amounts to the same slice of curriculum covered by a series of MMs won't produce these measurement shifts and will provide the long classic learning curve needed for decision making (see Figure 1.2).

A brief summary of the attributes for each type of measure is provided in Table 1.1.

I HAVE NEVER SEEN CBM BEING USED. IF IT'S SO GREAT, WHY ISN'T IT MORE POPULAR?

There are probably several reasons. We think the main one is that, until recently, the general education community hasn't been asking the kinds of questions CBM answers, but that has changed. Part of the change is because of increased professional and legislative emphasis on accountability, and part of it is because of the popularity of the Dynamic Indicators of Basic Early Literacy Skills (DIBELS). DIBELS started out as the application of CBM to early literacy skills, the same skills that were later given significance by the National Reading Panel (2000) and National Research Council (1998) reports. By the time those reports came out, the DIBELS measures had been administered to literally millions of students in general education, particularly within the context of state-level reading improvement initiatives (e.g., Reading First programs).

There has been some debate about whether or not DIBELS is CBM. For the most part, it seems accurate to say that DIBELS applies CBM procedures to early reading

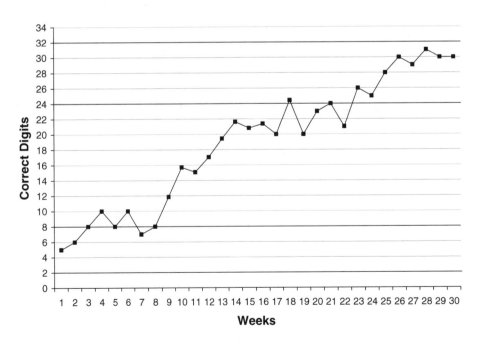

FIGURE 1.2. Example of a GOM or SBM progress-monitoring profile.

TABLE 1.1. Comparison of the Three Types of CBMs

General outcome measures (GOMs)	Skills-based measures (SBMs)	Mastery measures (MMs)
Primary uses		
• Screening • Survey-level testing • Progress monitoring	• Screening • Survey-level testing • Progress monitoring	• Diagnostic evaluation • Specific-level testing • To target content areas of concern • To target different proficiency levels and response types
Structure		
• Uses global/interactive tasks • Separate skills are not isolated or marked • Targets long-term goals • Often includes common classroom tasks	• Composed of mixed items drawn from a set of goals • Skills are usually sampled across a whole year's curriculum • Separate skills may be isolated or marked • Items are often cross-referenced to goals	• May only test one specific skill or short-term instructional objective • A large sample of performance is collected on each skill • Items are referenced to skills and/or proficiency levels • Some skills may be examined in isolation
Advantages		
• Provides perspective • Gives an overall impression of skill level • Useful for monitoring • No measurement shifts • Illustrates retention and generalization	• Gives an overall impression of skill level • Useful for monitoring • Illustrates retention • No measurement shifts	• Useful for double checking a problem indicated on a GOM or SBM • Useful for checking hypotheses about missing skills or subskills • Provides focus
Disadvantages		
• Provides little diagnostic information • Doesn't provide information about specific skills • Often includes a high proportion of items that are either above or below the student's skill level • Some content areas don't have convenient capstone tasks	• Small sample for each goal limits diagnostic utility • Often includes a high proportion of items that are either above or below the student's skill level • May not require generalization or interactive use of the skill	• Don't provide the big picture (no generalization or application) • Skill–subskill relationships may not be real • Can't be used for progress monitoring

tasks; however, there are differences in some scoring rules and item formats. Other modifications have also evolved with the development of web-based CBM management systems such as AIMSweb and Edcheckup. Most of these changes seem to fall under the heading of fine-tuning and are probably to be expected as the application evolves for new populations and content areas.

It is still true that many educators haven't heard of CBM, and there is an interesting reason for that: No one has advertised it. In a way, CBM is the people's measurement technology. Because it uses a set of administration and scoring rules that can be applied to a variety of materials, including tasks from a school's existing instructional materials, CBM does not require users to purchase test manuals and consumable test booklets (this book can serve as your test manual). Because there is very little for publishers to sell, CBM has not been advertised, marketed, and promoted the way traditional tests have. This means that you don't get junk mail pushing CBM in your mailbox at work—so far.

IS CBM USED IN SPECIAL EDUCATION OR GENERAL EDUCATION?

CBM was originally used in special and remedial education because its ability to target specific skills and its sensitivity to instruction make it particularly useful for adjusting instruction to individual student needs, but special educators really aren't the only ones who do that. As mentioned, the use of CBM by general educators has been growing. As also mentioned, everyone has become increasingly aware of the need to screen and progress monitor students in order to catch those who are falling behind as soon as possible. It is particularly important to progress monitor in high-impact content like reading, oral language, written expression, math, and social skills (as you'll find, not all of these areas are covered in this book). As a result, CBM is being increasingly adopted by whole school districts (and states) as a system for use with all students.

WHO GIVES CBM MEASURES?

It depends on why the measures are being given. Often CBMs are used three or four times over the course of the year to screen or benchmark all students by looking at their level of performance and rate of progress in key skills like reading, math, and written expression. The reading comprehension, math, and written expression measures can all be group administered. If you are well prepared, math and written expression (depending on the grade level of the students) take from 5 to 10 minutes each. Oral reading requires individual administration and, if the flow of students and materials is managed smoothly, one person should be able to collect three individual reading samples from a student in another 5 minutes. The process takes, at most, 20 minutes of actual student testing time. Most of that time will be in group-administered activity. For the reading, because all students in a school are being tested during screening/benchmarking, the actual administration is usually conducted by a team of general education teachers, special education teachers, school psychologists, reading specialists, and teaching assistants. We do not recommend using community contacts such as parents, volunteers, or peers.

Time spent preparing materials, organizing the space, and training people in how to administer, score, and record will pay off. Once all the testing is done, the data are then entered into a computer or web-based management system by someone on the school staff (again, not community volunteers). In Chapter 9, we provide a guide for setting up and managing these and more related activities.

Giving CBMs for the purpose of analyzing learning problems is a different matter. This book really is not about diagnostic testing. Testing for diagnostic purposes is usually carried out by someone who is an expert in the content area of concern as well as curriculum-based evaluation (CBE). This person could be a general education teacher, special education teacher, content-area specialist, or school psychologist. When CBMs are given for analysis of a learning problem, there is no standard set of tests. Instead, specific measures are selected to check on the presence or absence of those skills suspected to be causing the problem. In order to do this, we need to have a set of these measures available, but unfortunately, there are not any such complete sets of measures. There are a few resources for developing or identifying such materials, and these are provided in Box 2.1 of Chapter 2.

Finally, CBM is also used to monitor the effectiveness of instruction by giving the students repeated measures of the same skills over time in order to see trends in their learning.

IF I WANT TO USE CBM, DOES THIS MEAN I'LL NEED TO MAKE TESTS OUT OF THE INSTRUCTIONAL MATERIALS I'M USING?

This is an important question and is an issue of some debate. The answer depends on the answer to another question that would seem to be fairly basic for people interested in CBM—namely, "What is the definition of *curriculum*?" We have said that curriculum is "what you teach," meaning it is the standards that must be met for students to achieve social and academic competence, but some people define curriculum to include "how you teach" (meaning the teaching materials being used).

If you take the "how" view, the curriculum is not just the skills that are taught, but also the approach through which they are being taught. Therefore, you would want program-specific measures. (For example, if your reading materials used numerous illustrations, you would have illustrations on your reading CBM.)

If you take the "what" view of curriculum, you don't need to have tests using the same formats and examples as the instructional materials. You would be able to choose from already available generic measures. We subscribe to the "what" view. Here are some reasons for our position:

1. *Instructional programs don't follow the same sequences and schedules.* One of the biggest challenges in education is that what is taught and when it is taught really is not standardized across schools. It certainly is not standardized across published instructional programs. Obviously, this creates major problems in a mobile society. Therefore, measures that match one program won't necessarily work for other programs.
2. *Program-specific tests may not tell you if the learning has generalized.* Our particular opinion is that you should carefully review and select the curriculum and then measure skills without being bound to any particular set of instructional materials.

In fact, some may actually prefer to use CBM items that are somewhat different or at least mixed, to try to ensure that learning has generalized (you don't want a student who can only work problems that are presented in a certain format).

3. *Program-specific tests will make the teacher dependent on the program.* Instructional materials do not remain constant. They are often revised, or teachers select new ones. If teachers use program-specific tests, they will have to produce new ones every time a new program is selected.

WHERE DO I GET CBM MATERIALS?

There are many sources of CBM materials. Some must be purchased, and others are free. There are also materials that can be accessed on the web. Materials for the content areas addressed in this book will be referenced in those chapters. Just remember that when you construct or select materials for CBM, you must have these two things:

1. *Alignment:* The materials must match the task and outcomes. This means the materials you select must sample the content you are interested in (e.g., reading) and call for the student to produce the same skills you are teaching (e.g., reading orally).

2. *Adequate sampling:* Be sure there are enough items and that the time interval is long enough to allow the student the opportunities needed to display her knowledge. A good sample of behavior is necessary to make decisions about what a student knows.

Also remember that there is more to evaluation than giving a test. You have to score it properly, record the data accurately, and interpret them correctly. This book will give you information about CBM scoring rules and the interpretation of scores. Assessment is carried out to inform decision making; we need to know what the scores mean in order to use them.

2

CBM for Assessment and Problem Solving

Educators are active problem solvers. They are constantly making decisions—the decisions that go into planning instruction and then the interactive decisions as those plans are adjusted, modified, and occasionally thrown out the window. The number of decisions made in an average school on any given day, given the mixture of age, content, and personalities found in classrooms, dwarfs the number made in any corporation (and we would argue that they are often more important). Making educational decisions is part of the work done in the context of a classroom, school, district, or state department of education, but the sort of decisions made will be different depending on the work being done in these different contexts. One specific difference among these contexts is the balance of administrative work and teaching work.

The most administrative work occurs at the state department and school district levels. Administrators usually don't deliver instruction; they support and manage its delivery by providing leadership while advocating for, coordinating, and evaluating services. Teaching work pertains directly to teaching and learning. To do a good job at either administrative or teaching work, people need to solve problems and make good decisions. To carry out these tasks, at least four things are necessary:

1. A process for solving problems;
2. An understanding of the way decision making works in your job;
3. Good data; and
4. Adequate resources.

WHAT DO I NEED TO KNOW
ABOUT EDUCATIONAL DECISION MAKING?

As much as we would like to, we really won't be covering everything you need to know about educational decision making in the next few pages. There are whole books on that topic (a couple we recommend are referenced in this chapter and others are listed in the Resources and Further Reading section). We will, however, cover the basics.

The first thing to understand is that, while you need good data to make good decisions, collecting good data doesn't guarantee anything. In other words:

- To make good decisions you need to think productively.
- To think productively you need good information.

so

- You must have good information to make good decisions!

Without good information (i.e., data) there won't be any good decisions (the "garbage in, garbage out" idea), but just collecting good information never helped anyone. You have to do something with the information. That is why, to understand CBM fully, you need to understand how it can be used to make decisions and solve problems.

The second thing to consider is that there are different kinds of decisions. Various models have been suggested for the classification of educational decisions. One model that has recently gained popularity is the framework that came with the passage of the Reading First legislation. Within this framework (which is not specific to reading), we design and implement evaluation around four specific program functions. This is accomplished by asking a question for each function and developing a measurement procedure and decision-making process to answer each question. The whole package includes:

TYPE 1: SCREENING/BENCHMARKING DECISIONS

- *Function:* To determine quickly if students are performing adequately and/or if they are at risk for future learning failure (and may need additional educational support).
- *Question:* "Which students are currently at risk for academic failure?"
- *Evaluation procedure:* An efficient procedure for assessing all students on key skills.
- *Note:* Because the need is to collect data that can be used to identify quickly students who are at risk, the results will only indicate the problem. They usually will not provide detailed guidance on how to correct it. Also, the use of the term at risk is used to mean that the screening/benchmarking has predicted that the student may not succeed without additional support. It does not imply that the student has some sort of disability or inherent limitation.

TYPE 2: PROGRESS-MONITORING DECISIONS

- *Function:* To ensure that instruction is working.
- *Question:* "Is the student making adequate progress toward important goals?"
- *Evaluation procedure:* A procedure is used that:
  1. Is directly aligned with what is being taught;
  2. Is sensitive to learning; and
  3. Can be given frequently.

  Ideally, this measure should also yield information that can be easily summarized and displayed on a chart or graph.
- *Note:* Progress monitoring may occur at the group level (as classes are screened/benchmarked three or four times a year) or for individual students. The frequency of monitoring should increase when a student is found to be experiencing a problem.

TYPE 3: DIAGNOSTIC DECISIONS

- *Function:* To develop an instructional plan in response to a significant problem.
- *Question:* "What and how should we teach this student?"
- *Evaluation procedure:* A personalized evaluation procedure that will allow the careful and systematic examination of a student's skills. This allows the selection of individual expectations and teaching approaches.
- *Note:* Diagnostic evaluation is reserved for those relatively rare instances when progress monitoring shows that various educational supports have not worked.

TYPE 4: OUTCOME DECISIONS

- *Function:* To determine and document the effectiveness of an educational program.
- *Question:* "Has this program been a success?"
- *Evaluation procedure:* A procedure is used that will supply the information needed to determine if program goals have been met.
- *Note:* Outcome decisions can be based on measures ranging from specific reading CBM passages to statewide high-stakes assessments. What tool you select depends largely on who you need to supply with the results.

CBM can contribute to making each of these four types of decisions. In this book, we focus primarily on how to do screening/benchmarking and progress monitoring. We will also mention when diagnostic evaluation may be needed and what kinds of tools you could use to carry it out.

Obviously, we think that curriculum-based measures are excellent tools for a variety of purposes; however (and this should be no surprise), advocates of other kinds of assessment tools would probably argue exactly the same thing. Therefore, the real question is "Which technology is the best for this purpose?" and that is a question usually followed by "As compared to what?"

Here are some attributes that any instructionally useful (that is our standard) measure/assessment should have. It should:

1. Be useful for *deciding "what" and/or "how" students need to be taught*;
2. Have *adequate reliability and validity* for the purposes used;
3. *Be standardized*, so we can judge the quality of a student's performance in relation to a target;
4. *Sample defined domains* of knowledge, content, and behavior so that we can tell what the student had to know and do to work the items;
5. Be *aligned with the curriculum* taught to the student;
6. *Collect an adequate sample* of behavior to allow us to draw conclusions with confidence;
7. *Use appropriate scoring rules* so that the results we get supply an accurate representation of the student's skills and knowledge;
8. Allow for the *collection of rate data* so that we can reach conclusions about the student's fluency as well as his accuracy; and
9. *Be easy to use* so it is efficient to administer and score (and all the instruction in the school doesn't have to be shut down for 2 weeks).

Every measure that we use does not need to have every one of these attributes as long as they are all covered within our total assessment package, but it really would be better if they all did because each of these nine attributes is important to instructional utility. As it happens, these are also the general characteristics of well-designed criterion-referenced tests (CRTs). In general, CBM uses CRTs, although norms may be established for particular purposes.

WHAT IS A CRITERION-REFERENCED TEST?

It is worth spending some time talking about criterion-referenced measures and how norm-referenced tests (NRTs) and criterion-referenced tests differ because some of their differences are related to instructional utility. Understanding ideas like curriculum alignment, correct level of difficulty, and adequate sampling—all of which come up when one contrasts NRTs and CRTs—will help you understand why curriculum-based measures are designed and used the way they are.

An NRT uses a test to sample the student's behavior and then allows the user to compare that behavior to a *norm* (see below) so that the meaning of the score can be interpreted. A CRT uses a test to sample the student's behavior and then allows the user to compare that behavior to a *performance criterion* so that the meaning of the score can be interpreted. The referents are different because the measures are used for different purposes: NRTs are given to see how a student is doing in relation to others; CRTs are given to see how proficient a student is at a task.

A *norm* is basically the distribution of scores obtained by giving a measure to a randomly selected sample of students. Therefore, the scores in the norm represent the group from which the sample of students was selected. A *criterion* is a score that represents a desired level of performance. This is the type of standard established for CRTs. Usually the criterion specifies the level at which the student passes the test, meaning he no longer needs active instruction on the skill (this doesn't mean it will never be mentioned again). Criteria are commonly set by selecting successful students or class graduates and testing them to find the level of performance demonstrated by those who are good at the target skill. Sometimes they are set through research to find the level of performance that predicts future success. The norm and the performance criterion are both types of *standards* and should be established through a standardization process. This means that criterion-referenced measures (including CBM measures) are no less *formal* than norm-referenced measures.

There are some important differences between CRTs and NRTs. Because an NRT is designed to compare students, to other students it is necessary that, when a group of students takes the test, its members get a range of scores. If everyone who took an NRT got the same score—17, for example—there would be no way to say who was a high performer and who was a low performer; they would all just have 17. Consequently, the primary purpose of a normative measure, which is to allow the user to distinguish among students, would be lost. Therefore, the authors of NRTs write their tests in ways that exaggerate the performance differences among students (i.e., promote variability in the scores). By doing so, they often decrease educators' ability to use the tests to make teaching decisions.

Here are some ways authors of NRTs make sure students don't all get the same score:

How Authors Promote Variability on NRTs

1. They put a range of items on the test, starting from very early skills and going to those that are advanced.

2. They exclude items from the test that most students pass or that most students fail because these do not do a good job of discriminating among students.

The Effect This Can Have on Educational Value

1. This produces a test that, for any student, has a large number of items that are either above or below his instructional level. As a result, much of his performance is on portions of the curriculum that are not currently relevant to his education.
   • CBM is aligned with instructional objectives, so it targets areas of current importance to the student.

2. Most students pass the items that most teachers find important and emphasize. This means that items that cover important content may actually be thrown off an NRT!
   • CBM, because it is curriculum-based, only includes items that match instructional goals.

3. Because the tests cover a wide range of difficulty, the authors can only include a few items for each skill (adding more items for each skill would make the test too long).

4. Many NRTs, particularly achievement measures, are designed to be group administered or machine scored. Therefore, they use identification response item formats (e.g., multiple choice).

3. This means the sample of information collected for each skill is inadequate.
   • CBM provides enough items to collect an adequate sample of the student's performance.

4. This can cause misalignment between the conditions of testing and the behaviors teachers expect of students in the classroom.
   • CBM uses the same types of items students encounter in class and requires them to make the same sorts of responses.

ARE CBMs STANDARDIZED TESTS?

The term *standardized* has two meanings: The first is that the test is given in a standard fashion, meaning that there are administration and scoring procedures set out for everyone to follow; the second is that a *standard* (the norms or performance criteria) has been established so scores can be interpreted in terms of a validated referent. The process of developing the standard that will be used for these comparisons is called standardization.

CBM meets both of these definitions of standardized. It comes with administration and scoring procedures that need to be followed (and will be provided in this text) and with standards, in the form of performance criteria or norms that can be used to allow interpretation. These will also be provided when available.

Most CBMs are criterion referenced. The criteria are the same ones found in curriculum standards or objectives. They have nothing to do with how well other students may or may not be performing. For example, if a student is in the fall of his fifth-grade year, he should read aloud from fifth-grade material at about 104 words correctly per minute with 97% accuracy or better. That criterion for oral reading specifies a desired level of performance even if the average student in class is only reading 65 words correctly per minute.

HOW RELIABLE AND VALID IS CBM?

We're glad you asked!

While some measures are more reliable or valid than others, all the measures presented in this book meet general standards for reliability and validity. Appendix A contains a table with a few of the most recent reliability and/or validity studies for each of the content areas presented in this book. It is far from an exhaustive list since there have been more than 100 studies on the reliability or validity of CBM.

There are some CBM measures that aren't presented in this book, but that doesn't mean that they aren't reliable or valid—it means we didn't have room for them. Since new CBMs are still under development in several areas, it's important that you as the consumer check out their reliability and validity to make sure that they're appropriate for you to use.

WHERE DO THEY GET THE PERFORMANCE STANDARDS USED IN CBM?

There are a couple of ways performance standards are established. The first is to employ an *exemplar sampling* approach, in which you carefully draw a sample of *successful students* (the exemplars) from the setting where the students you are teaching will be going (e.g., the sample for beginning sixth graders is end-of-the-year sixth graders). You don't pay attention to things like the proportion of high-income and low-income students, males and females, or Easterners and Westerners in the group because we do not hold different expectations according to things like sex, race, or accidents of birth. You do make sure the group is successful at the skill in question (not necessarily outstanding or exceptional, just successful). Then the students are tested and their scores are used to establish the standard.

Another common way to set performance criteria is to use *norm sampling*. This involves testing all students at the end of the school year (or three times during the year) and using the average scores at a grade level or some percentage of them as the target level of performance for that grade from then on. Valid representative national norms have been assembled on some CBM measures (particularly in the area of reading). Many school districts prefer to use local norms. The obvious danger with local norms is that, in some schools, the average level of reading skill may be inadequate. It probably makes more sense and is easier to randomly sample a small group of students from one's school and compare their scores to the norms that are already validated. If this comparison shows the school is similar to the established norms, then there is nothing to be gained by generating local norms. If the school seems lower, local norms might give a false impression of student proficiency.

A third way to set performance standards could be called a *predictive validity* model. This involves empirically or statistically determining the level of performance that reliably predicts successful performance on a different outcome measure, usually at a future date. For example, we might want to know how many words read correctly to expect at the beginning of second grade to predict who will earn a proficient score on the state's second-grade CRT (given at the end of the year). When performance standards are set this way, you should consider what is being predicted and if it is a skill or performance level one actually wants students to work toward and meet.

It is worth mentioning that the term *benchmarks* is also used to refer to this type of performance standard. Here, the term indicates a score and is used as a noun, while previously the term *screening/benchmarking* indicated collecting data and was used as a verb. Benchmarks are scores that have been determined to predict later success on related tasks. Therefore, they are appropriate criteria to use for current performance. The benchmark score, however, is not the highest score, or even the middle score, but rather the lowest score one would accept that would indicate a student is *not* at risk for future academic failure. Even if students were not performing at an acceptable level at the beginning of the year (when the class was screened/benchmarked), as long as they make progress that will take them to mastery by the end of the year, we can feel confident that they will be performing proficiently and will not be at risk for later academic difficulty.

HOW CAN CBM BE USED FOR SCREENING/BENCHMARKING?

Screening/benchmarking is typically carried out using GOMs or SBMs. It is applied to find students who are falling behind or who are at risk for academic failure. An ideal screening/benchmarking test is quick and easy to give. It doesn't need to provide much information. It only needs to be a good predictor of future success (or failure) in the content area it covers. If screening/benchmarking signals a problem or potential problem, the student is typically supplied with educational support and increased progress monitoring. In cases where the problem seems to be extreme, it may be decided that the student needs to be given a diagnostic evaluation immediately. Often, students who have this level of need will already be known. Diagnostic evaluation is usually reserved for these students and those who, according to progress monitoring, fail to respond to support.

With CBM, it is possible to take a quick look at the status of all students in a school or district at least three times a year. This is done in the way their vital signs (temperature, heart rate, blood pressure) might be quickly checked by a physician or nurse. This analogy, that CBM can be used to check certain key skills indicating a student's "academic health," has been popularized by Mark Shinn (1989). It is based on the idea that performance on some tasks, while not giving the information one would need to plan an intervention, can be used to indicate the strength of a student's skill within a curriculum domain. If the score is outside of the acceptable range, professionals are alerted to the existence of a problem requiring additional attention. Using CBM in this fashion is particularly appropriate because of its efficiency, sensitivity to learning, and direct relationship to learning outcomes.

CBM can be used to find two indicators of a problem: first, low *performance* (or level of performance) in a key skill area; and second, low *progress* (or rate of progress) in the acquisition of key skills. By *acquisition* we mean learning, as seen in changes of student performance over time. As long as sufficiently sensitive tools are used for screening/benchmarking, the presence or absence of these changes can be seen. This means screening/benchmarking should be repeated for all students several times a year, usually a minimum of three. After a student has taken the screening/benchmark measures, his scores are compared to both level of performance and rate of progress expectations to make screening/benchmarking decisions. In this system, it is actually possible to recognize a learning problem in a student who performs relatively well on the tests but is not making progress. Here is what this might look like: A student named Larry moves into a new school district and on the fall oral reading screening/benchmarking gets a fairly high score. When tested again, in the winter screening/benchmarking, Larry gets the same score. This means he has not made progress. While he is still a high performer relative to many of his peers, his peers have made progress; they are currently low performers making good progress, while he, at the winter benchmark, is a relatively high performer making no progress. Given this information, you would worry more about Larry than about the other students.

CBM allows us to examine learning in the form of progress data. We can collect the progress data because CBM is a direct measure of what is taught and can be used in a repeated measurement format. Other commonly used measures can't be employed this way. Again, oral reading fluency (which is a GOM for reading) is a good example of a screening/benchmarking task as it is quick (three 1-minute sessions per student) and reflects the integration of many separate reading skills. Therefore, three 1-minute timed oral readings can make an excellent screener for reading problems.

Screening Summary

- *Evaluation question:* "Which students are at risk for academic failure?"
- *Function:* Screening/benchmarking procedures are used to check all students in order to identify those needing extra help or alternate forms of instruction.
- *Procedure:* Check "vital signs." Use CBM data to sort students quickly according to their level of performance and rate of progress. Choose their current program, a new program, or additional diagnostic evaluation according to their needs.

HOW CAN CBM BE USED FOR PROGRESS MONITORING?

Our knowledge of educational programming has not evolved to the point where we can guarantee positive results from every teaching decision made (incidentally, neither has the knowledge level in psychology, law, medicine, finance, or government). Therefore, we need to monitor the effects of decisions and instruction to see if they are working. Continuous monitoring of student learning coupled with a set of formal instructional decision rules can greatly improve the effectiveness of instruction. In fact, it is one of the most powerful innovations that can be introduced in a classroom or school system.

We use progress monitoring to inform the decisions we make during the process of program implementation. This is true at any program level. Progress monitoring can inform adjustments in statewide literacy initiatives or the multiplication instruction of a single student; the principles are the same. To succeed, the progress-monitoring tool must be sensitive to the impact of the instruction being delivered. Translated into educational practice, this means educators need to monitor with a measure that responds to the small changes in behavior resulting from day-to-day learning. That is the only way to get the feedback needed to make timely adjustments in instruction. The monitoring tools used for instructional interventions must:

- Directly sample what is being taught;
- Get an adequate sample of behavior; and
- Allow for repeated administration.

While most CBMs conform to these criteria, we often switch back to the GOMs or SBMs used for screening/benchmarking when we monitor progress. This is because the purpose of our intervention is to improve the student's skills to the point that he would not have failed the original screening/benchmarking (and would never have been identified as someone needing support). In addition, GOMs and SBMs have the advantage of adding the broader perspective of complex tasks. For example, writing samples may be used to collect monitoring data for written expression because they reflect a cluster of related skills even though a student's instruction may only be focusing on one or two specific skills within that cluster. (Similarly, it is common to use reading passages from the end of the school year or even the beginning of the following year to monitor a student's reading acquisition. In this way you can see how the student is advancing toward proficiency in the most difficult material with which he will be expected to work.)

Finally, it is important to note again that the sensitivity of a progress-monitoring system does not depend entirely on the way the CBM measure functions each time it is given. It also depends on whether or not the measure can be given multiple times. As a general rule, the more frequently you measure (typically one or two times per week for CBM), the more sensitive your data set will be to the influence of your intervention and, of course, the more frequently you will be able to make data-based decisions about the quality of your program. CBM is designed for this sort of frequent use, whereas other types of measures can't be repeated without jeopardizing their validity. One reason CBM works this way is that, as you may recall from Chapter 1, it was originally designed specifically for progress monitoring.

Progress Monitoring Summary

- *Evaluation questions:* "Is our intervention working?" and "What changes should we make?"
- *Function:* To ensure that instruction is working; to signal when a change is needed and to guide adjustments in the program.
- *Procedure:* Use measures that reflect responses to instructional interventions or programs in terms of progress toward the acquisition of skills and meeting of standards.

As already explained, it is more important to see that students are adequately progressing through the curriculum than it is to require them to learn from any particular method. This leads to another basic principle of progress monitoring in education: There is no reason to monitor if we don't intend to make changes. If a student (or group) is not progressing adequately, it is the teacher's (or organization's) responsibility to try to find a new approach to the instruction of that skill. While screening/benchmarking and progress-monitoring measures may alert you to the need for a change, they will not always give you the information you need to decide what kind of change you should make.

When progress monitoring indicates that the student is learning, the logical thing to do is to stay with the current program. If the indications are that the student is not learning, this can signal the need for a diagnostic evaluation. Diagnostic evaluation is not the focus of this text, but it may be worth a few lines to show how CBM can fit into diagnostic work.

One of the most likely explanations for a student's failure to perform a task is that he is missing the necessary prior knowledge to succeed. To put it another way, this assumption states that the most likely reason a student can't do something is that he doesn't know how. Therefore, when targeting inquiry and measurement, the most important learner characteristic to examine is the student's prior knowledge. For example, if a student is having trouble reading his sixth-grade history text, you would target the skills needed to read that book. These skills should reside in the curriculum.

When conducting a diagnostic curriculum-based evaluation, you don't want to let your thinking stray from the prior knowledge hypothesis. If you do, you may end up targeting and testing things like learning aptitude, intelligence, cognitive processing characteristics, perceptual abilities, auditory discrimination, visual–motor integration, or even general achievement. These are not examples of the skills and knowledge that make up the curriculum. Most of them are constructs that have only a hypothetical and/or correlational relationship to the curriculum. Instead, tools such as the Multilevel Academic Skills Inventory (MASI) can help maintain the focus on prior knowledge. They can also help pinpoint what specific skills need to be taught in a logical scope and sequence.

In order to target measurement and problem solving in a curriculum-based paradigm, you need an understanding of the curriculum area and direct measures of the student's skills. This means that, while your knowledge of the curriculum will help you come up with the targets, you will need CBM to check the student's status and find out if he doesn't know the key prerequisite skills. This is why selection of a correct standard and analysis of existing knowledge is so important.

In a well-designed curriculum, essential prerequisite knowledge is located at lower levels in the skill sequences. When you conduct the inquiry, CBM is the best way to get a good handle on how well the student has mastered those prerequisites. The GOMs and SBMs used for screening/benchmarking often do not supply enough of a sample or the specific focus you need to allow this sort of analysis. Therefore, specific-level MMs designed to target particular skills are commonly used for the diagnostic function.

SO WHERE DO WE GO FROM HERE?

Our goal for the first two chapters of this book has been to answer some of the questions that are asked about CBM in general terms of the "whats" and "whys." For the rest of the book, we turn to the "hows," as in "How do I implement CBM?"

BOX 2.1. Internet CBM Resources

Intervention Central—CBM Warehouse
www.interventioncentral.org/htmdocs/interventions/cbmwarehouse.shtml

National Center on Student Progress Monitoring
www.studentprogress.org

Big Ideas in Beginning Reading
reading.uoregon.edu

Research Institute on Progress Monitoring
progressmonitoring.org

Further online resources on CBM are listed in Box 2.1. Chapters 3 through 7 each provide, for different areas of the curriculum, a rationale for using CBM, a list of materials needed and where to get those materials, directions and scoring procedures, how often it should be administered, how much time it will take to give and score, criteria for performance, how to write goals and objectives, and frequently asked questions. Chapter 8 will take you through the process and procedures to set goals and graph the data as well as describe how CBM fits into an RTI model. Chapter 9 provides a guide for how to use CBM, how to get it going, and how to sustain it. Appendix A offers a table of recent reliability and/or validity studies for CBM; Appendix B provides resources that can be photocopied and used while conducting CBM, including quick administration and scoring guides for each CBM skill covered in this book, two checklists for conducting CBM, and a graph to plot the data.

RESOURCES AND FURTHER READING

Howell, K. W., Hosp, J. L., Hosp, M. K., & Macconell, K. (in press). *Curriculum-based evaluation: Linking assessment and instruction.* New York: Sage.

Shapiro, E. S. (2004). *Academic skills problems: Direct assessment and intervention* (3rd ed.). New York: Guilford Press.

3

How to Conduct Reading CBM

OVERVIEW OF WHY TO CONDUCT READING CBM

Many students struggle with reading. Because of this and because it is critical to success in and out of school, it should be assessed often. Reading CBM provides a reliable and valid way to (1) identify students who are at risk for reading failure, (2) identify which students are not making adequate progress given the instruction they are receiving, (3) identify students' instructional level, and (4) identify which students need additional diagnostic evaluation. Over 25 years of research has shown that there is no other assessment that does these things as well as CBM. Most other reading assessments do not provide an account of fluency that allows us to determine how automatic students are at performing a task. Automaticity is important because it demonstrates the student has mastered the skill.

The two best reasons for conducting Reading CBM are (1) that it is easy and time efficient to administer and score and (2) that it provides educators with information that can be used to inform instruction. Different measures are used for early reading as compared to reading. Early reading (which is discussed in Chapter 4) consists of letter–sound fluency (i.e., pronouncing letter sounds aloud from a randomized page of letters for 1 minute) and word identification fluency (i.e., reading common words aloud from a list of words for 1 minute). Other tasks associated with early reading are those assessed by DIBELS, such as initial sound fluency, phoneme segmentation fluency, letter naming fluency, and nonsense word fluency—which are also discussed further in Chapter 4.

Reading CBM consists of oral reading fluency (i.e., reading aloud from a passage for 1 minute) and maze passage reading (i.e., reading a passage silently and restoring every seventh word that has been deleted and replaced with three words).

Each of these assessments provides a different score, but all scores are based on the number of items correct in a set amount of time. This reflects the student's accuracy and fluency on the task. This information provides a database for each student so that appropriate instructional decisions can be made in a timely manner. Table 3.1 indicates which

TABLE 3.1. Recommended Reading CBM Task by Grade and Time of Year

Grade	CBM task	Time of year
Kindergarten	Letter sound fluency (LSF)	LSF = fall, winter, and spring
Grade 1	Oral reading fluency (ORF) and/or word identification fluency (WIF)	ORF = winter and spring WIF = fall, winter, and spring *or* If < 10 on ORF, administer WIF at any time
Grade 2	ORF	ORF = fall, winter, and spring
Grade 3	ORF	ORF = fall, winter, and spring
Grade 4+	Mazes	Mazes = fall, winter, and spring

Note. Based on Fuchs and Fuchs (2004).

tasks are recommended for grades K–4+. The tasks listed for kindergarten and grade 1 are covered in detail in Chapter 4. The rest are covered in detail in this chapter.

Once you have identified which Reading CBM skills are most appropriate to use, the next step is to gather the materials you will need to conduct CBM. The first skill we address, oral reading fluency (ORF), is the most commonly used for Reading CBM. The reason it is so common is that it is a capstone task in reading. In order to read a passage of text aloud quickly and accurately, you need to use a variety of different literacy skills, including decoding, vocabulary, and comprehension (particularly accessing prior knowledge). This is what makes ORF a good predictor of future reading performance.

After we review the materials needed and the administration and scoring rules for ORF CBM, we provide the same information for Maze CBM. Maze CBM is actually a better predictor than ORF CBM of future reading performance for students in the higher grades (fourth or higher). In addition, it appears to have slightly better face validity than ORF for its relationship to comprehension (i.e., many people have trouble understanding the relationship between ORF and comprehension, but not the relationship between Maze and comprehension; a reason for this is probably that Maze is more similar to other comprehension measures than ORF is).

ORF CBM

Materials Needed to Conduct ORF CBM

1. Different but equivalent reading passages (student and teacher/examiner copies).
2. Directions for administering and scoring ORF CBM.
3. A writing utensil and clipboard.
4. A stopwatch or countdown timer that displays seconds.
5. A quiet testing environment to work with students.
6. An equal-interval graph or a graphing program to plot the data.

ORF CBM Reading Passages

The ORF passages should be different but equivalent in grade level and should include at least 200 words per passage. The reading skills represented should be ones the student is expected to master throughout the entire school year. Typically, the passages are from the end of the school year or even the beginning of the following year. While the passages should be different, they should all be of equivalent difficulty (e.g., at the same grade level). It is important that the passages be as close in difficulty as possible. The best way to accomplish this is to purchase generic passages that have been developed specifically for collecting ORF data. Sources for obtaining passages for each of the reading areas are listed in Box 3.1.

The first time any of the ORF CBM materials are administered to the student, three equivalent passages should be used whether you are going to be conducting screening/benchmarking, progress monitoring, or survey-level assessment. This should be conducted in one testing session, but it can occur across consecutive days if needed. We recommend doing it in one session to save set-up time and obtain a more accurate score. The median score of these three samples will be used to provide the first data point on the student's graph. After that, 20–30 different but equivalent passages will be used to monitor student progress in reading throughout the year.

BOX 3.1. Where to Find Premade Reading CBM Passages (ORF and Maze)

$ indicates there is a cost for the passages and/or graphing program.

🖥   indicates computerized administration available.

✍   indicates data management and graphing available.

AIMSweb (Pearson) $✍

Website: *www.aimsweb.com*

Phone: 866-323-6194

Address: Harcourt Assessment, Inc.
         AIMSweb Customer Service
         P.O. Box 599700
         San Antonio, TX 78259

Products: • ORF passages (30 progress monitoring, 3 benchmarking for grades 1–8), English and Spanish
          • Maze passages (30 progress monitoring, 3 benchmarking for grades 1–8)

(continued)

Dynamic Indicators of Basic Early Literacy Skills (DIBELS) ✍

Website: *dibels.uoregon.edu*

Products: • ORF passages (20 progress monitoring, 3 benchmarking for grades 1–6),
             English and Spanish

Edcheckup $🖥✍

Website: *www.edcheckup.com*

Phone: 952-229-1441

Address: Edcheckup
           7701 York Avenue South, Suite 250
           Edina, MN 55435

Products: • ORF passages (23 each for grades 1–5+)
           • Maze passages (23 each for grades 1–5+)

Intervention Central

Website: *www.interventioncentral.org*

Products: • ORF passages (progress monitoring and benchmarking premade
             and create your own for grades 1–6)

Project AIM (Alternative Identification Models)

Website: *www.glue.umd.edu/%7Edlspeece/cbmreading/index.html*

Products: • ORF passages (14 to 20 each for grades 1–4)

Vanderbilt University $ (copying and postage only)

Phone: 615-343-4782

Address: Lynn Fuchs
           Peabody #328
           230 Appleton Place
           Nashville, TN 37203-5721

Products: • ORF passages (30 each for grades 1–6)

Yearly Progress Pro (CTB/McGraw-Hill) $🖥✍

Website: *www.ctb.com/mktg/ypp/ypp_index.jsp*

Phone: 800-538-9547

Products: • Maze passages (23 for grade 1, 33 for grades 2–8)

ORF CBM must be administered individually. Two copies of each passage will be needed. The student should have a copy of the ORF CBM passage in front of her, and the teacher/examiner should have a copy of the ORF CBM passage to write on, a timer, writing utensil, and the directions in front of him. See Figures 3.1 and 3.2 for examples of each type of passage. Note that the teacher/examiner's passage (Figure 3.2) has a running word total at the end of each line. This makes scoring much more efficient.

Directions and Scoring Procedures for ORF CBM

ORF CBM is used more than any other CBM skill area. Therefore, there are more materials available as well as multiple directions for administration and scoring. Below, we provide as examples two sets of administration directions from two different sources. Only one set of scoring criteria is provided since these do not deviate as much as the administration directions. It is important to use the same set of directions each time and

Pack Your Bags   Student Copy

"We're going on a trip!" said Dad when we sat down for
breakfast. "We only have two days to get ready. Everyone
will have to help out"

"Where are we going?" asked Sarah.

"We're going to the city," Dad answered.

"What city?" asked Anthony.

"Boston," said Dad. "It will take us about three hours to
drive there by car. There is a lot you can learn about our country's
past in Boston. Now, let's start planning."

Dad gave us each a bag and told us to pack enough clothes
for three days. Since it was summer, we didn't have to worry
about coats and boots. When Dad checked Sarah's bag he said
she should take a dress incase we went someplace fancy.

When he checked my bag he said, "Don't forget your
toothbrush!" He got to Anthony's bag and found it full of toys.
"Anthony, where are your clothes?" He helped him decide
which toys to leave behind so he could fit some clothes in the
bag.

That night, we talked about our trip. "Where will we stay
when we get to Boston?" I asked.

"We'll stay in a hotel right across from Copley Square,"
said Dad.

FIGURE 3.1. Example of student ORF CBM passage. Reprinted from Edcheckup (2005). Copyright 2005 by Children's Educational Services, Inc., and Edcheckup, LLC. Reprinted by permission.

Pack Your Bags

Examiner Copy

"We're going on a trip!" said Dad when we sat down for	12
breakfast. "We only have two days to get ready. Everyone	22
will have to help out."	27
"Where are we going?" asked Sarah.	33
"We're going to the city," Dad answered.	40
"What city?" asked Anthony.	44
"Boston, said Dad. "It will take us about three hours to	55
drive there by car. There is a lot you can learn about our	68
country's past in Boston. Now, let's start planning."	76
Dad gave us each a bag and told us to pack enough clothes	89
for three days. Since it was summer, we didn't have to worry	101
about coats and boots. When Dad checked Sarah's bag he said	112
she should take a dress incase we went someplace fancy.	123
When he checked my bag he said, "Don't forget your	133
toothbrush!" He got to Anthony's bag and found it full of toys.	145
"Anthony, where are your clothes?" He helped him decide	154
which toys to leave behind so he could fit some clothes in the	167
bag.	168
That night, we talked about our trip. "Where will we stay	179
when we get to Boston?" I asked.	186
"We'll stay in a hotel right across from Copley Square,"	196
said Dad.	198

Words Correct _____

Words Incorrect _____

FIGURE 3.2. Example of teacher/examiner ORF CBM passage. Copyright 2005 by Children's Educational Services, Inc., and Edcheckup, LLC. Reprinted by permission.

within a school or district if the data will be used to make comparisons across classrooms, grades, or schools. Changing the directions can change how the student performs on the task and, therefore, should be avoided. For your convenience, Appendix B includes a reproducible version of the directions and scoring rules for ORF CBM.

Directions for ORF CBM—Version 1[1]

1. Place the copy of the student passage in front of the student.
2. Place the teacher/examiner copy on the clipboard so the student cannot see it.
3. Say: ***"When I say 'Begin,' start reading aloud at the top of the page. Read across the page*** (point to the first line of the passage). ***Try to read each word. If***

---

[1]Adapted from Shinn (1989).

you come to a word you don't know, I'll tell it to you. Be sure to do your best reading. Do you have any questions? Begin." (*Trigger stopwatch or timer for 1 minute.*)

4. Follow along on the teacher/examiner copy as the student reads and put a slash (/) through any incorrect words.
5. At the end of 1 minute, say *"Thank You"* and mark the last word read with a bracket (]).

Directions for ORF CBM—Version 2[2]

1. Place the copy of the student passage in front of the student.
2. Place the teacher/examiner copy on the clipboard so the student cannot see it.
3. Say: *"I would like you to read this story aloud for me. Please start here (point to the first word on the student's copy) and read aloud. This is not a race. Try each word. If you come to a word that you do not know, you may skip it and go to the next word. You may start when I say 'Begin.' You may stop when I say 'Stop reading.' Do you have any questions? Begin."* (*Trigger stopwatch or timer for 1 minute.*)
4. Follow along on the teacher/examiner copy as the student reads and put an X through any incorrect words.
5. At the end of 1 minute, say: *"Stop reading"* and mark the end of the last word read with a slash (/).

Scoring ORF CBM

1. Count the total number of words attempted in 1 minute.
2. Count the total number of errors.
3. Subtract the total number of errors from the total number of words attempted to obtain the words read correctly (WRC) score.

SCORED AS CORRECT

- A word must be pronounced correctly, in accordance with the context of the sentence.
  Example: For the sentence *He will read the book* the word *read* must be pronounced "reed."
    o Read as: "He will *read* the book."
      Scored as: 5 WRC
    o Read as: "He will *red* the book."
      Scored as: 4 WRC

---

[2]Adapted from Edcheckup (2005).

- Repetitions: Words said over again are ignored.
    Example: *Bill jumped high.*
    ○ Read as: "Bill jumped . . . jumped high."
    Scored as: 3 WRC
- Self-corrections: Words misread initially but corrected within 3 seconds are scored as correct.
    Example: *The dog licked Kim.*
    ○ Read as: "The dog *liked* . . . (2 seconds) . . . licked Kim."
    Scored as: 4 WRC
- Insertions: If the student adds extra words, those words are counted neither as correct nor as errors.
    Example: *The big dog ran home.*
    ○ Read as: "The big *black* dog ran home."
    Scored as: 5 WRC
- Dialect/articulation: Variations in pronunciation explainable by local language norms or speech sound production are correct.
    Example: *I need a pen to sign my name.*
    ○ Read as: "I need a *pin* to sign my name."
    Scored as: 8 WRC

SCORED AS ERRORS

All errors are marked with a slash (/).

- Mispronunciations/word substitutions: Words either mispronounced or substituted with other words are errors.
    Example: *The house was big.*
    ○ Read as: "The *horse* was big."
    Scored as: The house was big. (3 WRC)
    Example: *Mother went to the store.*
    ○ Read as: "*Mom* went to the store."
    Scored as: Mother went to the store. (4 WRC)
- Omissions: Each word omitted is an error.
    Example: *Juan went to a birthday party.*
    ○ Read as: "Juan went to a party."
    Scored as: *Juan went to a birthday party.* (5 WRC)
- Hesitations: When a student hesitates to pronounce a word correctly within **3 seconds**, the student is told the word and an error is scored.
    Example: *Leslie is moving to Miami.*
    ○ Read as: "Leslie is moving to MmmIiiiAaa . . . (3 seconds)" [Provide the word *Miami* and mark it as an error.]
    Scored as: *Leslie is moving to Miami.* (4 WRC)
- Reversals: When a student transposes two or more words, those words not read in the correct order are errors.
    Example: *The fat cat walked past us.*

     o Read as: "The cat fat walked past us."
      Scored as: *The f̶a̶t̶ c̶a̶t̶ walked past us.* (4 WRC)

SPECIAL SCORING EXAMPLES

- Numerals: Numbers are counted as words and must be read correctly within the context of the passage.
  Example: *August 6, 2003*
  - Read as: "August six, two thousand-three"
    Scored as: 3 WRC
  - Read as: "August six, two zero zero three"
    Scored as: *August 6, 2̶0̶0̶3̶* (2 WRC)
- Hyphenated words: Each morpheme separated by a hyphen(s) is counted as an individual word if it can stand alone.
  - *Son-in-law* (3 WRC)
  - *Forty-five* (2 WRC)
  - *bar-b-que* (1 WRC)
  - *re-evaluate* (1 WRC)
- Abbreviations: Abbreviations are counted as words and must be read correctly within the context of the sentence (e.g., Mrs., Dr.).
  - *Dr., Mrs., Ms., Mr.* (1 WRC each)
  - Should be read as: "doctor, missus, miz, mister"
  - **Not** "D-R, M-R-S, M-S, M-R."

SPECIAL ADMINISTRATION AND SCORING CONSIDERATIONS FOR ORF CBM

1. If the student reads fewer than 10 words correctly in 1 minute, do not administer additional passages at the same level. (See procedure for survey-level assessment below).
2. The student is not corrected if she misreads a word. The only time you provide the correct word is if she hesitates for 3 seconds.
3. If the student skips a row, you draw a line through it and do *not* count it in the scoring as attempted or errors.
4. If the student finishes in less than 1 minute, note the number of seconds it took to complete the passage and prorate the score. The formula for prorating is:

$$\frac{\text{Total number of words read correctly}}{\text{Number of seconds to read the passage}} \times 60 = \text{Estimated number of words read correctly in 1 minute}$$

Example: The student finished reading the passage in just 54 seconds and got 44 words correct.

$$\frac{44}{54} \times 60 = .815 \times 60 = 48.9$$

We estimate that the student would have read approximately 49 words correctly in 1 minute had we provided more words and timed her for the full 1 minute.

MAZE CBM

Similar to the information provided for ORF CBM, this section provides a review of the materials needed and the administration and scoring rules for Maze CBM. We have also included an example of two sets of administration directions from two different sources. Just as with ORF CBM, it is important to use the same set of directions each time within a school or district if the data will be used to make comparisons across classrooms, grades, or schools. Changing the directions can change how the student performs on the task and, therefore, should be avoided.

Materials Needed to Conduct Maze CBM

1. Different but equivalent Maze passages (student and teacher/examiner copies).
2. Directions for administering and scoring Maze CBM.
3. A writing utensil and clipboard.
4. A stopwatch or countdown timer that displays seconds.
5. A quiet testing environment to work with students.
6. An equal-interval graph or a graphing program to plot the data.

Maze Reading Passages

The reading passages should be different but equivalent in level of difficulty and should include at least 300 words and 42 deleted words (with three replacement words each). The reading skills should represent the skills the student is expected to master by the end of the school year. While the passages should be different, they should all be of equivalent difficulty. The best way to accomplish this is to purchase generic passages that have been developed specifically for this purpose. Sources for obtaining passages for each of the reading areas are listed in Box 3.1.

The first time any of the Reading CBM materials are administered to the student(s), three equivalent passages should be used whether you are going to be conducting screening/benchmarking, progress monitoring, or survey-level assessment. This should be conducted in one testing session, but it can occur across consecutive days if needed. We recommend doing it in one session to save set-up time and obtain a more accurate score. The median score of these three samples will be used to provide the first data point on the student's graph. After that, 20–30 different but equivalent passages will be used to monitor student progress in reading throughout the year.

Maze passages can be administered to a group. The students should each have a copy of the Maze CBM passage in front of them, and the teacher/examiner should have a copy of the administration directions and a timer. To score the passages, the teacher/examiner will also need the examiner copy of the Maze passage with the answers (see Figures 3.3 and 3.4 for an example of each) and a writing utensil. Scoring can be facilitated by making a transparency of a correctly scored passage. This transparency can then be placed over the student's work for rapid error recognition.

Name _____   Date _____

The Visitor   Student Copy

Tap, tap, tap. I was reading a book. But (**I, top, bit**) kept hearing a noise at the (**red, eat, window**). Tap, tap. I began reading again. (**Clunk, Top, Ball**) scrape, tap, tap. I looked out (**stick, of, sit**) the window. It was dark outside. (**I, Did, A**) couldn't see anything. I looked back (**tick, pit, at**) my book. It was hard to (**so, find, and**) my place. I found it and (**it, began, tree**) to read. I heard the noise (**up, again, into**). This time I was not going (**bad, to, an**) stop reading. I didn't want to (**hit, tip, lose**) my place again.

Clunk, scrape, scrape. (**I, Dig, Ran**) had to look up again. I (**lip, nap, was**) mad. I knew I had lost (**stop, my, jump**) place. I just had to find (**map, out, tan**) what was making that noise on (**din, the, still**) window. I walked to the door. (**I, At, Six**) turned on the outside light. Tap, (**scrape, hill, back**). I stepped outside to look at (**blue, the, what**) window. There it was—a big (**June, walk, sit**) bug. It kept flying against the (**in, who, window**) again and again. Now I knew (**rip, too, I**) had a visitor. I didn't need (**sip, to, live**) stop to check it out again, (**you, ping, so**) I just went back to my (**its, up, reading**).

Correct _____
Incorrect _____

FIGURE 3.3. Example of student maze CBM passage. Copyright 2005 by Children's Educational Services, Inc., and Edcheckup, LLC. Reprinted by permission.

The Visitor   Examiner Key

Tap, tap, tap. I was reading a book. But (**I,** top, bit) kept hearing a noise at the (red, eat, **window**). Tap, tap. I began reading again. (**Clunk,** Top, Ball) scrape, tap, tap. I looked out (stick, **of,** sit) the window. It was dark outside. (**I,** Did, A) couldn't see anything. I looked back (tick, pit, **at**) my book. It was hard to (so, **find,** and) my place. I found it and (it, **began,** tree) to read. I heard the noise (up, **again,** into). This time I was not going (bad, **to,** an) stop reading. I didn't want to (hit, tip, **lose**) my place again.

Clunk, scrape, scrape. (**I,** Dig, Ran) had to look up again. I (lip, nap, **was**) mad. I knew I had lost (stop, **my,** jump) place. I just had to find (map, **out,** tan) what was making that noise on (din, **the,** still) window. I walked to the door. (**I,** At, Six) turned on the outside light. Tap, (**scrape,** hill, back). I stepped outside to look at (blue, **the,** what) window. There it was—a big (**June,** walk, sit) bug. It kept flying against the (in, who, **window**) again and again. Now I knew (rip, too, **I**) had a visitor. I didn't need (sip, **to,** live) stop to check it out again, (you, ping, **so**) I just went back to my (its, up, **reading**).

FIGURE 3.4. Example of teacher/examiner Maze CBM passage. Copyright 2005 by Children's Educational Services, Inc., and Edcheckup, LLC. Reprinted by permission.

Directions and Scoring Procedures for Maze CBM

We provide two sets of administration directions for Maze CBM to reflect how it would be conducted if (1) you were using practice items, or (2) you were providing the directions without practice items. For your convenience, Appendix B includes a reproducible version of the directions and scoring rules for Maze CBM.

Directions for Maze CBM with Practice Items[3]

1. Place a copy of the student passage with the *practice items* in front of each student (see Figure 3.5 for an example of the practice items).
2. Say: *"Today I want you to read a short story. The story you will read has some places where you will need to choose the correct word. Read the story. When you come to three words in dark print, choose the word that belongs in the sentence.*

   "We will do some examples. Look at the first page. Read the sentence. The sentence says: 'Bill threw the ball to Jane. Jane caught the (dog, bat, ball).' *Which one of the three words belongs in the sentence?"*
3. After the students respond, say: *"The word* ball *belongs in the sentence 'Bill threw the ball to Jane. Jane caught the ball.' Circle the word* ball.*"*
4. *"Now let's try sentence number 2. Read the sentence. The sentence says: 'Tom said, "Now you* (jump, throw, talk) *the ball to me."' Which of the three words belongs in the sentence?"*
5. After the students respond, say: *"The word* throw *belongs in the sentence 'Now you throw the ball to me.' Circle the word* throw.*"*
6. Place a copy of the student passage in front of each student face down.
7. Say: *"Now you are going to do the same thing by yourself. You will read a story for 1 minute. When I say 'Stop,' stop reading. Do not begin reading until I tell you to start. Whenever you come to three words that are in dark print, circle the word that belongs in the sentence.*

   "Choose a word even if you're not sure of the answer. At the end of 1 minute, I will say 'Stop.' If you finish early, check your answers. Do not go on to the next page. You may turn your paper over and begin when I say 'Start.' Are there any questions?

   "Remember to do the best you can. Pick up your pencils. Ready? Start."
   (Trigger stopwatch or timer for 1 minute.)
8. Walk around the room to monitor that students are only circling one word per set and not skipping around the page.
9. At the end of 1 minute, say: *"Stop. Put your pencils down."*
10. Separately administer two more passages using the following directions.
11. Say: *"Now you will do the same thing with another story. Remember to choose the word that belongs in the sentence. Choose a word even if you're not sure of*

---

[3]Adapted from Edcheckup (2005).

Name _____ Date _____

Maze Procedure
Student Practice Examples

1. Bill threw the ball to Jane. Jane caught the (**dog, bat, ball**).

2. Tom said, "Now you (**jump, throw, talk**) the ball to me."

FIGURE 3.5. Maze CBM practice item. Copyright 2005 by Children's Educational Services, Inc., and Edcheckup, LLC. Reprinted by permission.

      the answer. You may begin when I tell you to." (*Trigger stopwatch or timer for 1 minute.*)

12. At the end of 1 minute, say: *"Stop. Put your pencils down."*
13. Collect all the student sheets.

Directions for Maze CBM without Practice Items[4]

1. Place a copy of the student passage in front of each student face down. (It is helpful to have the student's name already on the sheet before starting.)
2. Say: *"When I say 'Begin,' turn to the first story and start reading silently. When you come to a group of three words, circle the one word that makes the most sense. Work as quickly as you can without making mistakes. If you finish the page, turn the page and keep working until I say 'Stop' or you are all done. Do you have any questions? Begin."* (*Trigger stopwatch or timer for 3 minutes.*)
3. Walk around the room to monitor that students are only circling one word per set and not skipping around the page.
4. At the end of 3 minutes, say: *"Stop. Put your pencil down and turn your sheet over."*
5. Collect all the student sheets.

Scoring Maze CBM

1. Count the total number of responses attempted in 3 minutes, or whatever time period is specified by for the materials you are using (other common time limits are 1 minute or 2½ minutes).
2. Count the total number of errors.
3. Subtract the total number of errors from the total number attempted to obtain the Words Correctly Restored (WCR) score.

_____

[4]Adapted from AIMSweb (Shinn & Shinn, 2002b).

SCORED AS CORRECT

- Correct word must be circled or underlined.
  - The big dog (**slept**, **ran**, **can**) fast.
  - The big dog (**slept**, **ran**, **can**) fast.

SCORED AS ERRORS

- If the incorrect word is circled, underlined, or left blank, you mark the correct choice with a slash (/).
  - The (**turtle**, **boy**, **pulls**) has a little tail.
  - The (**turtle**, **boy**, **pulls**) has a little tail.
  - The (**turtle**, **boy**, **pulls**) has a little tail.

SPECIAL ADMINISTRATION AND SCORING CONSIDERATIONS FOR MAZE CBM

1. Scoring is discontinued if three consecutive errors are made. If three consecutive responses are incorrect, then you do not count or score any of the responses following the three consecutive incorrect.
2. If the student finishes before 3 minutes, write the number of minutes and seconds on the student's sheet and prorate her score. The formula for prorating is:

$$\text{Step 1:} \frac{\text{Total number of seconds}}{\text{Number of correct answers}} = \text{Calculated value}$$

$$\text{Step 2:} \frac{\text{Total number of seconds in \_\_ minutes}}{\text{Calculated value}} = \text{Estimated total correct}$$

Example: The student finished the Maze passage in 2 minutes and 30 seconds (150 seconds) and got 40 WRC.

$$\text{Step 1:} \frac{150}{40} = 3.75$$

$$\text{Step 2:} \frac{180}{3.75} = 48 \text{ estimated total correct}$$

We estimate that the student would have correctly restored 48 words in 3 minutes had we provided more words and timed the student for the full 3 minutes. (*Note:* 180 is the total number of seconds in 3 minutes. If you need to prorate for a scale that uses a different time interval, convert the number of minutes to seconds.)

3. The same directions are used for group and/or individual administration.

HOW OFTEN SHOULD ORF AND MAZE CBM BE GIVEN?

So far, we have explained how to administer and score the Reading CBM measures to get performance data. Next, we want to find out how to use CBM to get progress-monitoring data. To do this you will need to give the measures several times. Therefore, just as important as knowing *how* to give the measures is knowing *when* to give them. The information provided here will be reviewed in each subsequent content chapter.

It is recommended that all students be screened/benchmarked at least three times a year in order to examine both their level of performance and rate of progress in important skill areas. As you'll recall, performance data are collected at one point in time but progress-monitoring data are seen by giving the CBM measures repeatedly across time. Screening/benchmarking typically occurs once per quarter and would include testing in the fall, winter, and spring. Special considerations for screening/benchmarking include testing at the appropriate time. For example, we do not recommend screening/benchmarking students during the first 2 weeks of school for two reasons:

- Students often need instruction to recapture some skills they may have forgotten.
- Not all students may have enrolled or started to attend school. This means early screening/benchmarking may miss some students who need help. Also, teachers may be reassigned based on final enrollment figures.

Screening too early might cause you to overidentify students who appear to need additional instructional help. This can affect the use of resources and take valuable time and instruction away from those students who need it most. Therefore, we recommend waiting at least 2 weeks after the start of school to screen/benchmark all students and avoiding winter and spring screening/benchmarking dates that follow long breaks.

Using the screening/benchmarking data, we can identify which students' progress should be monitored. More frequent progress monitoring is recommended for those students who are most at risk for academic failure. This can be conceptualized in most cases as those performing in the bottom 25% of the class on the screening/benchmarking measures, or any student who is considered at risk based on norms or benchmark criteria. This group will often include students with disabilities as well as students who are merely behind their same-grade peers. Because these students are already behind, it is critical to monitor their progress often and consistently. By "often," we mean at least once per week; twice per week would be optimal. By "consistently," we mean using CBM assessments that are at the same difficulty level. If the criterion changes from week to week, we cannot determine if the student is making adequate progress given the instruction she is receiving. Producing multiple versions of passages that are of equivalent difficulty can be very difficult and time consuming. This is why we recommend purchasing commercial materials that reduce variability. Monthly progress monitoring of all students can provide information about the effectiveness of classroom instruction.

The last point on how often to administer CBM assessments relates to survey-level assessment (SLA). SLA refers to a CBM technique that provides a general sample of the student's behavior and is typically used to find a student's instructional level and help guide instruction. This is most helpful when a student is new to a school or teacher. SLA can also be conducted along with screening/benchmarking since you already will have collected three samples of student work. These three samples can be used as the first three data points. The use of SLA has only been tested on ORF CBM and Math CBM (Computation). Therefore, it is not addressed in each subskill area. For those areas in which it does apply, we provide information on how to conduct it.

HOW MUCH TIME DOES IT TAKE TO ADMINISTER AND SCORE READING CBM?

The time needed to score each student passage is the same for ORF and for Maze CBM regardless of grade level. For ORF CBM, once the student is in front of the teacher/examiner, the time it takes to give the directions, have the student read for 1 minute, and score the passage is 2–3 minutes total. If you are screening/benchmarking and giving three passages at one time, it should take 5–6 minutes total. You will also need to factor in time for the student to move to where the teacher/examiner is, whether that is in the same room or down the hall. Obviously, it makes more sense to go to the students rather than have the students come to the examiner as one way to save time. Another way to save time is to have everything printed out and ready to go with the students' names already indicated on the appropriate forms. One way to do this is to print labels.

For Maze CBM, once the student is in front of the teacher/examiner, the time it takes to give the directions, have the student read for 3 minutes, and score the passage is 4–5 minutes total. If you are screening/benchmarking and giving three passages at one time, it should take 12–15 minutes total. While students in older grades may make more restorations, this should not increase the time needed to score the passage. One way to save time is to have an overlay with the correct answers on it that the teacher/examiner can place over the Maze passage. All the teacher/examiner would have to do is count the number of errors and subtract this from the total attempted. Remember that ORF CBM must be given individually but that Maze CBM can be given to a whole class. So the time to administer it to a group would be the same, but you would need to add 20–30 seconds to score each student's passages.

EXPECTED GROWTH RATES AND NORMS FOR ORF AND MAZE CBM

How Much Progress Can We Expect in Reading?

Just as it is important to know from where the student is starting, it is equally important to know how much progress we can expect the student to make given typical instruction. These rates of progress are often referred to as growth rates. In order to determine growth rates, researchers have measured typically developing students and assessed what their rate of progress is on ORF and Maze CBMs (Fuchs, Fuchs, Hamlett, Walz, & Germann, 1993). See Table 3.2 for ORF CBM growth rates and Table 3.3 for Maze CBM growth rates. It is important to note that these growth rates do not imply that students are learning a set number of new words per week. The growth rates for ORF CBM, for example, provide an indication of the average number of words per week we would expect stu-

TABLE 3.2. Weekly Growth Rates for ORF CBM: Words Read Correctly (WRC)

Grade	Realistic growth rates per week (WRC)[a]	Ambitious growth rates per week (WRC)[a]	Growth rates per week (WRC)[b]
1	2	3	1.80
2	1.5	2	1.66
3	1	1.5	1.18
4	0.85	1.1	1.01
5	0.5	0.8	0.58
6	0.3	0.65	0.66

[a]Data from Fuchs et al. (1993).
[b]Data from Deno, Fuchs, Marston, and Shin (2001).

dents to improve by if they are continuing to learn and improve in reading. These are not necessarily new words they are reading. Instead, on average, the students are reading the same words but at a faster rate each week when we assess their performance.

It is important to understand that these normative growth rates certainly do not represent the maximum progress possible. Progress beyond these levels can be expected when instruction is carefully designed and implemented. In fact, higher levels must be expected in those cases where students are behind in a skill area and must be caught up.

These progress expectations, like any other form of standard, are used as a criterion against which student behavior can be compared. When a student's behavior (i.e., actual progress) does not meet the standard (i.e., expected growth rate), it is our obligation to find a way to fix that problem. We might do this by building up a prerequisite skill, increasing the length of daily lessons, or altering the way we respond when an error is made. We would *not* do it by lowering the expectation. Learning is the result of instruction, so when the rate of learning is inadequate, it doesn't always mean there is something wrong with the student. It does mean the instruction needs to be changed to better meet the student's needs.

TABLE 3.3. Weekly Growth Rates for Maze CBM: Words Correctly Restored (WCR)

Grade	Ambitious growth rates per week (WCR)
1	0.4
2	0.4
3	0.4
4	0.4
5	0.4
6	0.4

Note. Data from Fuchs and Fuchs (2004).

Proficiency Levels or Benchmarks for Reading CBM

In addition to having a standard to which to compare a student's weekly growth (i.e., her rate of progress), it is important to have standards for level of performance. These are often referred to as benchmarks. Benchmarks here are actual scores, whereas the screening/benchmarking referred to earlier is the act of assessing. Benchmarks are helpful because they are predictive of later student achievement. Good, Gruba, and Kaminski (2002) have investigated the level of proficiency students need to attain on ORF CBM in order to be successful on other types of reading assessments, typically high-stakes assessments. This is helpful for teachers because it allows them to determine who is on track and who needs additional assistance to be successful at reading. The benchmark scores we provide in Table 3.4 are from the DIBELS website. The benchmark scores provide the lowest score we would accept that would indicate a student is *not* at risk for future academic failure.

Norms for Reading CBM

Another way to set standards for performance is to compare a student's score to the performance of others in her grade or at her instructional level. These norms have been collected over numerous years and from numerous sources. It should be mentioned that they have not been collected in a traditional sense, making sure that the students in the norm group have similar characteristics to the U.S. population as determined using the U.S. Census. It is interesting to note, however, that the data have been collected on thousands of students across the country, and the numbers are very similar. This adds credibility to the idea that these norms provide a good indication of how students perform. Norms are typically collected at three different points throughout the year, in the fall, winter, and spring, allowing educators to have a better idea of how their students are performing in regard to level of performance and rate of progress during three different times of the year instead of only being able to make comparisons at one point in the year (see Chapter 2 for a further discussion). Table 3.5 provides norms for ORF CBM, and Table 3.6 provides norms for Maze CBM.

TABLE 3.4. Benchmarks for ORF CBM: Words Read Correctly (WRC)

| Grade | DIBELS (2006) | | |
	Fall (WRC)	Winter (WRC)	Spring (WRC)
1	—	20	40
2	44	68	90
3	77	92	110
4	93	105	118
5	104	115	124
6	109	120	125

TABLE 3.5. Norms for ORF CBM: Words Read Correctly (WRC)

Grade	Percentile	AIMSweb (2008)[a]			Hasbrouck & Tindal (2006)		
		Fall (WRC)	Winter (WRC)	Spring (WRC)	Fall (WRC)	Winter (WRC)	Spring (WRC)
1	90%	56	84	113	—	81	111
	75%	25	52	85	—	47	82
	50%	**9**	**26**	**56**	**—**	**23**	**53**
	25%	3	14	31	—	12	28
	10%	0	7	17	—	6	15
2	90%	107	133	148	106	125	142
	75%	82	108	123	79	100	117
	50%	**57**	**81**	**97**	**51**	**72**	**89**
	25%	29	56	71	25	42	61
	10%	14	27	46	11	18	31
3	90%	135	153	167	128	146	162
	75%	107	130	143	99	120	137
	50%	**80**	**100**	**115**	**71**	**92**	**107**
	25%	51	72	86	44	62	78
	10%	31	44	56	21	36	48
4	90%	153	170	186	145	166	180
	75%	123	143	159	119	139	152
	50%	**101**	**116**	**129**	**94**	**112**	**123**
	25%	75	91	102	68	87	98
	10%	49	63	75	45	61	72
5	90%	171	185	199	166	182	194
	75%	146	161	174	139	156	168
	50%	**114**	**130**	**145**	**110**	**127**	**139**
	25%	87	100	112	85	99	109
	10%	61	74	85	61	74	83
6	90%	184	198	211	177	195	204
	75%	160	171	184	153	167	177
	50%	**133**	**145**	**157**	**127**	**140**	**150**
	25%	104	116	128	98	111	122
	10%	72	85	97	68	82	93
7	90%	187	196	208	180	192	202
	75%	163	172	185	156	165	177
	50%	**136**	**144**	**157**	**128**	**136**	**150**
	25%	108	116	127	102	109	123
	10%	85	90	100	79	88	98
8	90%	185	192	201	185	199	199
	75%	166	171	182	161	173	177
	50%	**143**	**148**	**158**	**133**	**146**	**151**
	25%	114	119	130	106	115	124
	10%	84	89	100	77	84	97

[a]2008 data updated for third printing.

TABLE 3.6. Norms for Maze CBM: Words Correctly Restored (WCR)

		AIMSweb (2008)[a]		
Grade	Percentile	Fall (WCR)	Winter (WCR)	Spring (WCR)
1	90%	8	13	18
	75%	3	7	12
	50%	**1**	**3**	**7**
	25%	0	1	3
	10%	0	0	1
2	90%	13	21	25
	75%	8	16	19
	50%	**4**	**10**	**14**
	25%	2	6	9
	10%	0	3	5
3	90%	21	25	27
	75%	16	19	21
	50%	**11**	**14**	**15**
	25%	7	9	10
	10%	3	6	7
4	90%	22	31	33
	75%	17	25	26
	50%	**12**	**18**	**19**
	25%	8	13	13
	10%	5	8	9
5	90%	27	32	36
	75%	21	26	30
	50%	**16**	**20**	**24**
	25%	10	14	17
	10%	7	10	12
6	90%	31	38	41
	75%	25	31	32
	50%	**19**	**24**	**25**
	25%	13	17	18
	10%	8	11	12
7	90%	33	36	42
	75%	27	29	34
	50%	**20**	**22**	**26**
	25%	14	16	18
	10%	10	12	13
8	90%	34	33	40
	75%	27	26	32
	50%	**20**	**20**	**25**
	25%	15	15	19
	10%	11	11	14

[a]2008 data updated for third printing.

SURVEY-LEVEL ASSESSMENT WITH ORF CBM

Another use of ORF CBM is SLA. This doesn't mean surveys like the annoying ones conducted by telemarketers in the middle of dinner. Here the word *survey* means that we are taking a broad look at the student's performance—we're surveying it. SLA is used to find a student's instructional level in reading (currently it is only available to use with ORF since there has not been much work done with proficiency levels of Mazes). This provides a starting point for instruction as well as a more accurate level of materials to use for monitoring the student's progress.

The first step is to administer three separate passages at the student's grade level and find the median WRC and median errors. These can be recorded on the SLA sheet for ORF CBM. A reproducible version of this form is available in Appendix B. The student's median scores are then compared to the performance criteria and drawn on the graph. If both the WRC and errors are within the instructional range, this is the student's instructional level. Curriculum materials should be at this level and the level of materials used to progress monitor should be related to that level (using the chart in the bottom right to select the appropriate level). If the student's performance falls in the frustrational range (i.e., below the instructional level), administer three passages from the next lowest level. For example, if the first passages were at a third-grade level and the student's median WRC was 50 with a median of 7 errors, select three passages at the second-grade level and administer them to the student. Continue this process until the student's performance is within the instructional range. If you find that the student's performance is in the frustrational range on first-grade-level materials, you should switch to Early Reading CBM materials. The instructions for SLA are included on the reproducible sheet in Appendix B.

HOW TO USE THE INFORMATION
TO WRITE READING IEP GOALS AND OBJECTIVES

CBM data are an excellent source for writing goals and objectives. Because educators can monitor how well the student is doing on a weekly basis, they no longer have to hold their breath and hope that when they test her at the end of the year she will have reached her goal(s). CBM is the best measurement system currently available to monitor students' progress toward long-term goals. The best part about using CBM to monitor progress is that it is so sensitive to student improvement that if the student is learning the material, you will see an increase in her CBM score each week. The reverse also holds true: If the student is not learning the material, you will not see an improvement each week. This allows teachers to make instructional changes as often as needed. Using CBM in this way stacks the cards in the student's favor to reach the goal and objectives the team has developed.

In addition, CBM is extremely efficient to use for writing goals and objectives because it provides a way to clearly define and observe the behaviors we are most interested in. For reading, these behaviors are saying letter sounds, reading words, and reading passages. Correctly restoring missing words is the behavior for comprehension.

Therefore, incorporating CBM information into writing goals and objectives provides clear and straightforward criteria on which one can gauge students' success. This is accomplished by clearly defining and including the following seven components:

1. *Time* (the amount of time the goal is written for, typically 1 year)
   • "In 1 year . . . "
2. *Learner* (the student for whom the goal is being written)
   • " . . . Jose will . . . "
3. *Behavior* (the specific skill the student will demonstrate)
   • " . . . read aloud . . . "
4. *Level* (the grade the content is from)
   • " . . . second-grade . . . "
5. *Content* (what the student is learning about)
   • " . . . reading . . . "
6. *Material* (what the student is using)
   • " . . . passage from ORF CBM progress-monitoring material . . . "
7. *Criteria* (the expected level of performance, including time and accuracy)
   • " . . . 90 words correctly in 1 minute with greater than 95% accuracy."

Procedures for setting criteria are provided in Chapter 8.

EXAMPLE OF GOALS

• ORF goal
  ○ In one year, Edgar will read aloud a second-grade passage from ORF CBM progress-monitoring material at 90 WRC in 1 minute with greater than 95% accuracy.
• Maze goal
  ○ In 30 weeks, Devin will correctly restore missing words on a fourth-grade Maze passage from Maze CBM progress-monitoring material at 20 WCR in 3 minutes with greater than 95% accuracy.

The same principles apply to writing objectives, but one should use a shorter time frame.

EXAMPLE OF OBJECTIVES:

• ORF objective
  ○ In 10 weeks, Edgar will read aloud a second-grade passage from ORF CBM progress-monitoring material at 50 WRC in 1 minute with greater than 95% accuracy.
• Maze Objective
  ○ In 10 weeks, Devin will correctly restore missing words on a fourth-grade Maze passage from Maze CBM progress-monitoring material at 8 WCR in 3 minutes with greater than 95% accuracy.

FREQUENTLY ASKED QUESTIONS ABOUT READING CBM

1. *For ORF CBM, should I have students read the title on the page or should I read it to them?* You should *not* have the student read the title nor should you read it to her. It is not counted in the total words for the passage and may give the students some background information. Remember, this is a time to assess, not teach. If you come across a set of materials that includes the words in the title in the total word count for the passage (or in the directions), you should have the student read them (we are not currently aware of any, but you never know what you'll find).

2. *For ORF CBM, what happens if I start the stopwatch and the student starts reading silently?* You should stop the student. Get a different passage at the same difficulty level, remind her that she needs to read aloud so that you can hear her, and start over, including reading the directions.

3. *For ORF CBM, what if the student does not read the first word in 3 seconds?* You should say the word, put a slash through it, and continue to have the student read, keeping the timer going all along.

4. *If the student is not making good progress, should I lower the goal?* No. The first step should be to determine what skill(s) the student is missing that is preventing her from making progress, teach those skills, and continue to monitor her progress. If you don't know what skill(s) to teach, you may need to give a diagnostic evaluation, such as using mastery measures.

5. *How long do I have to wait to raise the goal if the student is performing better than I thought she would?* After collecting at least six to eight data points, if the student has four *consecutive* data points above the goal line, then it should be raised.

6. *Can I make my own ORF CBM passages, or do I have to purchase them?* We recommend that you purchase them to save time and to ensure that they are all of equivalent difficulty level, but you could make your own passages.

7. *How much training does it typically take to learn how to do ORF and Maze CBM?* We have found that after practicing with seven to ten students, people are typically very good at conducting CBM.

8. *Why do some of the scores on the norms drop from the spring to the fall of the next grade?* The material being read is at a higher level of difficulty (the next grade level), so you would expect a student to score lower on more difficult material.

9. *Can I change the directions or how I score the passages?* No. These measures were researched using the standardized procedures we have provided. If the directions or scoring criteria are changed, then the measure is changed, and we do not know what the reliability and validity are.

10. *Do ORF or Maze CBM passages come in languages other than English?* Yes. Many publishers of CBM passages have Spanish versions (ORF more so than Maze). We have indicated this in Box 3.1 on where to obtain materials.

11. *Can I use benchmark scores on ORF CBM to put students in instructional groups?* Yes, if you have students with similar instructional needs. These groups should be flexible, and students should be evaluated and regrouped every 6–8 weeks.

12. *Not everyone in my class is on the same instructional level. Should I still give them all the same ORF or Maze CBM passages?* All students should be screened/benchmarked on their grade level; however, students should be progress monitored on their instructional level—especially if they are receiving instruction on that level. The best way to handle this is to give both the grade-level and the instructional-level passages each week so that you have an indication of how students are doing given the instruction they are receiving (instructional level) and how well it is transferring to more difficult passages (grade level).

13. *What should I do with the scored passages?* This information can be kept in a portfolio along with the graphed data to demonstrate progress over the year.

14. *I only have 20 ORF or Maze passages, but I need to progress monitor for 35 weeks. Is it OK to use the same passages again?* Yes. Once you have used all 20, start using them again. The student probably doesn't remember specific items she did 20 weeks ago. This also means that you should not use the passages as homework or additional practice if you want to use them again.

RESOURCES AND FURTHER READING

Bean, R. M., & Lane, S. (1990). Implementing curriculum-based measures of reading in an adult literacy program. *Remedial and Special Education, 11*(5), 39–46.

Bradley-Klug, K. L., Shapiro, E. S., Lutz, J., & DuPaul, G. J. (1998). Evaluation of oral reading rate as a curriculum-based measure within a literature-based curriculum. *Journal of School Psychology, 36,* 183–197.

Fuchs, L. S., Fuchs, D., Hosp, M. K., & Hamlett, C. L. (2003). The potential for diagnostic analysis with curriculum-based measurement. *Assessment for Effective Intervention, 28*(3/4), 13–22.

Hintze, J. M., Daly, E. J., & Shapiro, E. S. (1998). An investigation of the effects of passage difficulty level on outcomes of oral reading fluency progress monitoring. *School Psychology Review, 27,* 433–445.

Scott, V. G., & Weishaar, M. K. (2003). Curriculum-based measurement for reading progress. *Intervention in School and Clinic, 38,* 153–159.

Shinn, M. R., & Shinn, M. M. (2002). *AIMSweb training workbook: Administration and scoring of reading curriculum-based measurement (R-CBM) for use in general outcome measurement.* Eden Prairie, MN: Edformation.

4

How to Conduct Early Reading CBM

OVERVIEW OF WHY TO CONDUCT EARLY READING CBM

Students who have mastered certain early reading skills (e.g., identifying letter sounds, reading basic words) in kindergarten and first grade are much more likely to continue on the road to becoming successful readers. Those students who have not mastered these early reading skills by kindergarten and first grade are at risk of continuing to fall further and further behind their peers and not becoming good readers. The research on early intervention tells us that the chances of helping students become proficient readers is greatly increased the earlier one intervenes. Waiting until second or third grade stacks the deck against teachers, making it much more difficult to help these students become proficient readers. The good news is that we know we can teach these important early reading skills and change the trajectory of these students' achievement in reading.

Using the Early Reading CBM measures can assist educators in determining who is at risk early on so that intervention and progress monitoring can start right away. Just like Reading CBM, measures used for Early Reading CBM also provide a way to identify which students are not making adequate progress given the instruction they are receiving so that appropriate instructional changes can be made. This is possible because the information provides a database for each student so that instructional decisions can be made in a timely manner. These measures require the student to be accurate as well as fluent, allowing one to determine how automatic students are at performing a task. Remember, automaticity is important because it represents a higher level of skill mastery.

Early Reading CBM consists of letter sound fluency (LSF) and word identification fluency (WIF). As mentioned in the previous chapter, there are other tasks associated with early reading like those assessed by the DIBELS, which include initial sound fluency, phoneme segmentation fluency, letter naming fluency, and nonsense word fluency.

These tasks are worth considering if you are interested in students' skills in phonemic awareness. We will briefly describe these skills and encourage people to look at the DIBELS measures on the web, as they are available to download for free along with all of the administration and scoring procedures used with the DIBELS measures. We will spend more time discussing LSF and WIF, however, neither of which is included in DIBELS. Similar to the reading tasks covered in the previous chapter, each of these tasks, including the DIBELS measures, provides a different score; each score is based on the number of items correct in a set amount of time to reflect the student's accuracy and fluency with the task.

Once you have identified which CBM skill to use, the next step is to gather the materials you will need to conduct CBM. First, we address DIBELS by providing a brief overview of each task. Next, we address LSF CBM in detail by reviewing the materials needed and the administration and scoring rules. Last, we provide this same detailed information for WIF CBM.

OVERVIEW OF DIBELS MEASURES

Initial Sound Fluency and Phoneme Segmentation Fluency

Initial sound fluency (ISF) and phoneme segmentation fluency (PSF) are the two DIBELS measures designed to assess phonological awareness. ISF requires the student to identify and produce the first sound/phoneme in a word. PSF requires the student to produce all of the individual sounds/phonemes (initial, medial, and end) he hears in words.

Initial Sound Fluency

The student is shown a page with four pictures. The teacher/examiner names each picture and asks the student to recognize and produce the first sound in a word the teacher/examiner says aloud. For example, if the four pictures were a boat, fork, dog, and ladder, the student would be asked, "Which picture begins with /d/?" To be marked correct, the student must either point to the picture of the dog or say *dog*. This task is timed on how long it takes (in seconds) to respond to a total of 16 prompts, producing an accuracy and fluency score for the number of correctly identified and produced initial phonemes.

Phoneme Segmentation Fluency

The teacher/examiner reads aloud a list of two-, three-, four-, and five-phoneme words (e.g., *as, hat, stop, points*), and the student is asked to produce all the sounds in the word— for example: "Tell me the sounds in *cat*." The student would need to respond /k/ /a/ /t/ to receive three credits, one for each phoneme. This task is timed for 1 minute as the teacher/examiner reads a list of words and the student produces the correct phonemes, providing an accuracy and fluency score for the number of correctly produced individual phonemes.

Nonsense Word Fluency

Nonsense word fluency (NWF) is the DIBELS measure designed to assess decoding skills. NWF provides an indication of how well students can map the correct sounds/phonemes onto letters/graphemes. This skill provides a clear understanding of how well students can use their basic decoding skills to read short vowel sounds and consonants.

The student is shown a page with 50 short nonsense words two or three letters in length. The teacher/examiner tells the student, "Point to each letter and tell me the sounds *or* read the whole word." Examples of what the words look like are: *tif, ot, sup, kef*. To receive credit, the student must either produce the correct individual sounds (e.g., /t/ /i/ /f/) or read the whole word (e.g., *tif*). Either response would be scored three correct letter sounds. This task is timed for 1 minute as the student reads the rows of words, providing an accuracy and fluency score for the number of correctly produced letter sounds.

Letter Naming Fluency

Letter naming fluency (LNF) does not assess phonological awareness or decoding; rather, it is used as a risk indicator for reading. This task is similar to other rapid naming tasks that do not use letters but instead ask the student to quickly name colors, numbers, or objects.

The student is shown a page of upper- and lower-case letters in random order. The teacher/examiner tells the student, "Point to each letter and tell me the name of that letter." This task is timed for 1 minute as the student reads the rows of letters, providing an accuracy and fluency score for the number of correctly produced letter names.

While LNF can be used as a risk indicator, it may be more efficient to use the LSF CBM task. We want students to be able to name the letters, but the skill that is more closely related to decoding and reading is knowing the *sounds* of the letters. Given the choice, we encourage teachers to use LSF CBM, which is described in detail below.

LSF CBM

Materials Needed to Conduct LSF CBM

1. Different but equivalent reading sheets (student and teacher/examiner copies).
2. Directions for administering and scoring LSF CBM.
3. A writing utensil and clipboard.
4. A stopwatch or countdown timer that displays seconds.
5. A quiet testing environment to work with students.
6. An equal-interval graph or a graphing program to plot the data.

LSF CBM Reading Sheets

LSF reading sheets should have different items (or sequences of items) and should have at least 26 letters per sheet. The best way to accomplish this is to purchase or obtain generic sheets that have been developed specifically for collecting LSF data. Sources for obtaining these sheets are listed in Box 4.1.

BOX 4.1. Where to Find
Premade Early Reading CBM Sheets and Lists (LSF and WIF)

$ indicates there is a cost for the sheets or lists and/or graphing program.
🖳 indicates computerized administration available.
✎ indicates data management and graphing available.

AIMSweb (Pearson) $✎

Website: *www.aimsweb.com*

Phone: 866-323-6194

Address: Harcourt Assessment, Inc.
           AIMSweb Customer Service
           P.O. Box 599700
           San Antonio, TX 78259

Products: • LSF (30 progress monitoring sheets, 3 benchmarking sheets),
             English and Spanish

Edcheckup $✎

Website: *www.edcheckup.com*

Phone: 952-229-1441

Address: Edcheckup
           7701 York Avenue South, Suite 250
           Edina, MN 55435

Products: • LSF (23 sheets)
           • WIF (23 sheets)

Intervention Central ✎

Website: *www.interventioncentral.org*

Products: • WIF (1 list per grade K–3 English, 1–2 Spanish)

Project AIM (Alternative Identification Models)

Website: *www.glue.umd.edu/%7Edlspeece/cbmreading/index.html*

Products: • LSF (12 sheets)

Vanderbilt University $ (copying and postage only)

Phone: 615-343-4782

Address: Lynn Fuchs
           Peabody #328
           230 Appleton Place
           Nashville, TN 37203-5721

Products: • LSF (10 sheets)
           • WIF (10 lists)

The first time LSF is administered to the student(s), three equivalent sheets should be used, whether you are conducting screening/benchmarking or progress monitoring. This should be conducted in one testing session, but it can occur across consecutive days if needed. We recommend doing it in one session to save set-up time and obtain a more accurate score. The median score of these three samples will be used to provide the first data point on the student's graph. After that, 20–30 different but equivalent sheets will be used to monitor student progress in reading throughout the year.

LSF must be administered individually. Two copies of the sheet will be needed. The student should have a copy of the LSF CBM sheet in front of him, and the teacher/examiner should have a copy of the LSF CBM sheet to write on, a timer, a writing utensil, and the directions. See Figures 4.1 and 4.2 for examples of each type of sheet.

Directions and Scoring Procedures for LSF CBM

For your convenience, Appendix B includes a reproducible version of the directions and scoring rules for LSF CBM.

Directions for LSF CBM[1]

1. Place the copy of the student sheet in front of the student.
2. Place the teacher/examiner copy on the clipboard so the student cannot see it.

t	d	n	r	p	c	z	v	w	k
m	b	t	f	v	z	i	c	d	p
v	y	e	l	b	j	s	t	f	a
c	n	f	r	m	b	t	h	z	s
j	k	p	s	f	h	i	r	o	m
s	z	p	i	j	r	e	d	g	o
j	g	a	t	s	h	c	r	k	l
j	u	k	y	a	s	z	e	i	v
m	s	d	g	f	l	b	v	j	c
t	e	m	l	w	j	y	z	f	v

FIGURE 4.1. Example of student LSF CBM sheet. Reprinted from AIMSweb (2003). Copyright 2003 by Edformation, Inc. Reprinted by permission.

---

[1]Adapted from AIMSweb (Shinn & Shinn, 2002a).

Given To: _____   Given By: _____   Date: _____

t d n r p c z v w k	/10 (10)
m b t f v z i c d p	/10 (20)
v y e l b j s t f a	/10 (30)
c n f r m b t h z s	/10 (40)
j k p s f h i r o m	/10 (50)
s z p i j r e d g o	/10 (60)
j g a t s h c r k l	/10 (70)
j u k y a s z e i v	/10 (80)
m s d g f l b v j c	/10 (90)
t e m l w j y z f v	/10 (100)

_____ / _____

FIGURE 4.2. Example of teacher/examiner LSF CBM sheet. Reprinted from AIMSweb (2003). Copyright 2003 by Edformation, Inc. Reprinted by permission.

3. Say: *"**Here are some letters** (point to the student copy). **Begin here** (point to the first letter) **and tell me the SOUNDS of as many letters as you can. If you come to a letter you don't know, I'll tell it to you. Are there any questions? Put your finger under the first letter. Ready? Begin."** (Trigger stopwatch or timer for 1 minute.)*
4. Follow along on the teacher/examiner copy as the student reads and put a slash (/) through any incorrect letters.
5. At the end of 1 minute say *"**Thank you**"* and put a bracket (]) after the last sound provided.

Scoring LSF CBM

1. Count the total number of letter sounds attempted in 1 minute.
2. Count the total number of errors.
3. Subtract the total number of errors from the total number of letter sounds attempted to obtain the total letter sounds correct (LSC) score.

SCORED AS CORRECT

A letter sound must be pronounced correctly, using the most common sound of the letter.

- Vowel sounds: Short vowel (not long vowel) sounds are considered correct. A most common sounds pronunciation key is provided in Table 4.1.

    Example: a, e, i, o, u
    - Read as: /a/ (like *apple*), /e/ (like *echo*), /i/ (like *itch*), /o/ (like *octopus*), /u/ (like *up*)

    Scored as: 1 letter sound correct (LSC) *each* (for a total of 5 LSC)
- Self-corrections: Sounds mispronounced initially but corrected within 3 seconds are scored as correct and *sc* is written above the letter.

    Example: a
    - Read as: long /a/ sound as in *ape* (2 seconds) . . . short /a/ sound as in *apple*

    Scored as: a̶ (1 LSC)

TABLE 4.1. Most Common Sounds Pronunciation Key

Letter	Example
a	apple
e	echo
i	itch
o	octopus
u	up
b	big
c	cat
d	dad
f	fat
g	go
h	hat
j	jump
k	kit
l	lip
m	mat
n	not
p	pat
q	quick
r	rat
s	sit
t	top
v	van
w	will
x	ox
y	yell
z	zip

- Dialect/articulation: Variations in pronunciation explainable by local language norms or speech sound production are correct.
  Example: s
  o Read as: /th/ instead of /s/ would be accepted if this is due to an articulation problem.
  Scored as: 1 LSC
- Added vowel or schwa sound: Sounds with the added "uh" sound are considered correct.
  Example: b, t, m
  o Read as: /buh/ /tuh/ /muh/
  Scored as: 1 LSC *each* (for a total of 3 LSC)

SCORED AS ERRORS

All errors are marked with a slash (/).

- Mispronunciations/letter sound substitutions: Letter sounds either mispronounced or substituted with other letter sounds are errors.
  Example: p
  o Read as: /b/
  Scored as: p̸ (0 LSC)
- Omissions: Each letter sound omitted is an error.
  Example: t, d, n, r, p, c, i, l
  o Read as: /t/ /d/ /n/ /p/ /c/ /i/ /l/
  Scored as: t, d, n, r, p, c, i, l (7 LSC)
- Hesitations: When a student hesitates to pronounce the sound correctly within **3 seconds**, the student is told the sound and an error is scored.
  Example: t, d, n, r, p, c, i, l
  o Read as: /t/ /d/ /n/ /r/ /p/ /c/ (hesitates 3 seconds on *i*). Say: "/i/." Point to next letter and say: **"What sound?"** /l/.
  Scored as: t, d, n, r, p, c, i̸, l (7 LSC)
- Reversals: When a student transposes two or more sounds, those sounds not read in the correct order are errors.
  Example: t, d, n, r, c, p, i, l
  o Read as: /t/ /d/ /n/ /c/ /r/ /p/ /i/ /l/
  Scored as: t d n r̸ c̸ p i l" (6 LSC)

SPECIAL ADMINISTRATION AND SCORING CONSIDERATIONS FOR LSF CBM

1. If the student says the letter *name* instead of the letter *sound*, say: **"Remember to tell me the sound the letter makes, not its name."** This is provided *one time* only.
2. If the student makes an error, he is not corrected. The only time a letter sound is provided is if the student hesitates for 3 seconds.

3. If the student skips a row, draw a line through it and do *not* count it in the scoring as attempted or as errors.

4. The capital letter *I* and lowercase *L* look alike, so either sound is considered correct.

5. If the student does not get any sounds correct in the first row, discontinue the task.

6. If the student finishes in less than 1 minute, note the number of seconds it took to complete the sheet/list and prorate the score. The formula for prorating is:

$$\frac{\text{Total number of sounds read correctly}}{\text{Number of seconds it took to read}} \times 60 = \text{Estimated number of letter sounds in 1 minute}$$

Example: The student finished the sheet in just 50 seconds and got 20 sounds correct.

$$\frac{20}{50} \times 60 = 0.40 \times 60 = 24$$

We estimate that the student would have read approximately 24 letter sounds correctly in 1 minute had we provided more letters and timed the student for the full 1 minute.

WIF CBM

Materials Needed to Conduct WIF CBM

1. Different but equivalent reading sheets (student and teacher/examiner copies).
2. Directions for administering and scoring WIF CBM.
3. A writing utensil and clipboard.
4. A stopwatch or countdown timer that displays seconds.
5. A quiet testing environment to work with students.
6. An equal-interval graph or a graphing program to plot the data.

WIF CBM Lists

The lists should have different items (or sequences of items) but be equivalent in difficulty (e.g., at the same grade level) and should consist of at least 50 words each. The reading skills should sample those the student is expected to master throughout the entire school year. The best way to accomplish this is to purchase generic sheets that have been developed specifically for this purpose. Sources for obtaining these sheets are listed in Box 4.1.

The first time any of the WIF CBM materials are administered to the student, three equivalent lists should be used, whether you are going to be conducting screening/

benchmarking or progress monitoring. This should be conducted in one testing session, but it can occur across consecutive days if needed. We recommend doing it in one session to save set-up time and obtain a more accurate score. The median score of these three samples will be used to provide the first data point on the student's graph. After that, 20–30 different but equivalent lists will be used to monitor student progress in reading throughout the year.

WIF must be administered individually. Two copies of the sheet will be needed. The student should have a copy of the WIF CBM sheet in front of him, and the teacher/examiner should have a copy of the WIF CBM sheet to write on, a timer, a writing utensil, and the directions. See Figures 4.3 and 4.4 for examples of each type of sheet.

Directions and Scoring Procedure for WIF CBM

For your convenience, Appendix B includes a reproducible version of the directions and scoring rules for WIF CBM.

Directions for WIF CBM[2]

1. Place the copy of the student list in front of the student.
2. Place the teacher/examiner copy on the clipboard so the student cannot see it.
3. Say: *"When I say 'Begin,' I want you to read these words as quickly and correctly as you can. Start here (point to the first word) and go down the page (run your finger down the first column). If you don't know a word, skip it and try the next word.*

Student: _____   Date: _____

Class: _____   Correct Items: _____

Total Items Attempted: _____

tell	first	write	before
don't	these	work	call
your	because	both	wash
sit	does	very	been
best	their	found	cold
its	those	goes	sing
green	many	right	or
wish	off	sleep	which

FIGURE 4.3. Example of student WIF CBM list. Reprinted from Intervention Central (2006).

[2]Adapted from Fuchs and Fuchs (2004).

Curriculum-Based Assessment List: Examiner Copy

This answer key contains 32 items from the following assessment list(s):

- *Dolch Words: Second Grade*

Student: _____ Date: _____

Class: _____ Correct Items: _____

Total Items Attempted: _____

Item 1 tell	Item 2 first	Item 3 write	Item 4 before	4/4
Item 5 don't	Item 6 these	Item 7 work	Item 8 call	4/8
Item 9 your	Item 10 because	Item 11 both	Item 12 wash	4/12
Item 13 sit	Item 14 does	Item 15 very	Item 16 been	4/16
Item 17 best	Item 18 their	Item 19 found	Item 20 cold	4/20
Item 21 its	Item 22 those	Item 23 goes	Item 24 sing	4/24
Item 25 green	Item 26 many	Item 27 right	Item 28 or	4/28
Item 20 wish	Item 30 off	Item 31 sleep	Item 32 which	4/32

FIGURE 4.4. Example of teacher/examiner WIF CBM list. Reprinted from Intervention Central (2006).

Keep reading until I say 'Stop.' Do you have any questions? Begin." *(Trigger stopwatch or timer for 1 minute.)*

4. Follow along on the teacher/examiner copy as the student reads and *put a slash (/) through any incorrect words.*

5. At the end of 1 minute, say: *"Stop"* and put a bracket ( ]) after the last word read.

Scoring WIF CBM

1. Count the total number of words attempted in 1 minute.
2. Count the total number of errors.
3. Subtract the total number of errors from the total number of words attempted to obtain the total words identified correctly (WIC) score.

SCORED AS CORRECT

- A word must be pronounced correctly to be scored as correct.
  Example: *made*
  ○ Read as: /made/ with a long /a/
  Scored as: 1 WIC
- Self-corrections: Words mispronounced initially but corrected within 3 seconds are scored as correct.
  Example: *where*
  ○ Read as: /were/ (2 seconds) . . . /where/
  Scored as: 1 WIC
- Dialect/articulation: Variations in pronunciation explainable by local language norms or speech sound production are correct.
  Example: *either*
  ○ Read as: /either/ with a long /i/ or long /e/
  Scored as: 1 WIC

SCORED AS ERRORS

- Mispronunciations/word substitutions: Words either mispronounced or substituted with other words are errors.
  Example: *mother*
  ○ Read as: /mom/
  Scored as: mother 0 WIC
- Omissions: Each word omitted is an error.
  Example: *and, as, at, one, said, into, could*
  ○ Read as: /and/ /as/ /one/ /said/ /into/ /could/
  Scored as: *and, as, at, one, said, into, could* 6 WIC
- Hesitations with no attempt to read word: When a student hesitates for **2 seconds**, the student is prompted to read the next word by pointing to it and saying **"What word?"**
  Example: *and, as, at, one, said, into, could*
  ○ Read as: /and/ /as/ /at/ (hesitates 2 seconds on *one*). Point to *said* and say: **"What word?"** /said/ /into/ /could/.
  Scored as: *and, as, at, one, said, into, could* 6 WIC
- Hesitations when sounding out a word: When a student is sounding out a word for **5 seconds**, the student is prompted to read the next word by pointing to it and saying **"What word?"**
  Example: *and, as, at, one, said, into, could*
  ○ Read as: /and/ /as/ /at/ /ooooonnnnnn/ (hesitates 5 seconds on *one*). Point to *said* and say **"What word?"** /said/ /into/ /could/.
  Scored as: *and, as, at, one, said, into, could* 6 WIC
- Reversals: When a student transposes two or more words, those words not read in the correct order are errors.

Example: *and, as, at, one, said, into, could*

    ○ Read as: /and/ /as/ /at/ /one/ /into/ /said/ /could/

      Scored as: *and, as, at, one, ~~said~~, ~~into~~, could* 5 WIC

SPECIAL ADMINISTRATION AND SCORING CONSIDERATIONS FOR WIF CBM

1. If the student makes an error, he is not corrected.
2. If the student skips a word, it is scored as an error.
3. If the student finishes in less than 1 minute, note the number of seconds it took to complete the word list and prorate the score. The formula for prorating is:

$$\frac{\text{Total number of sounds read correctly}}{\text{Number of seconds it took to read}} \times 60 = \text{Estimated number of words read correctly in 1 minute}$$

Example: The student finished the sheet in just 50 seconds and got 35 sounds correct.

$$\frac{35}{50} \times 60 = 0.70 \times 60 = 42$$

We estimate that the student would have read approximately 42 words correctly in 1 minute had we provided more words and timed the student for the full 1 minute.

HOW OFTEN SHOULD LSF AND WIF CBM BE GIVEN?

In Chapter 3, we provide additional details on how often and when to administer CBM for the different purposes of screening/benchmarking, progress monitoring, and survey-level assessment. Below we provide only an outline for screening/benchmarking and progress monitoring as survey-level assessment to find instructional levels has not yet been developed for LSF and WIF CBM. We suggest you refer to Chapter 3 for a more in-depth discussion on how often and when to give CBM for these different purposes.

-   Screening/benchmarking = all students in a classroom or grade level, once per quarter (three to four times per school year); typically conducted in the fall, winter, and spring.
-   Progress monitoring = students in the bottom 25% of the class based on the screening/benchmarking assessment, at least one time per week—preferably two times per week. This includes any student who is considered at risk based on norms or benchmark criterion.
-   Monthly progress monitoring of all students can provide information about the effectiveness of classroom instruction.

HOW MUCH TIME DOES IT TAKE
TO ADMINISTER AND SCORE EARLY READING CBM?

The time needed to score each student sheet is the same for LSF and WIF CBM. Once the student is in front of the teacher/examiner, the time it takes to give the directions, have the student read for 1 minute, and score the sheet is 2–3 minutes total. If you are screening/benchmarking and giving three sheets at one time it should take 5–6 minutes total. As indicated in Chapter 3, you will also need to factor in time for the student to move to where the teacher/examiner is, whether that is in the same room or down the hall. Obviously, it makes more sense to go to the students rather than have the students come to the examiner as one way to save time. Another way to save time is to have everything printed out and ready to go with the students' names already indicated on the appropriate forms. One way to do this is to print labels.

EXPECTED GROWTH RATES AND NORMS FOR LSF AND WIF CBM

Proficiency Levels or Benchmarks for Early Reading CBM

Unlike ORF and Maze CBM, there is currently no research on realistic or ambitious growth rates for LSF and WIF CBM, but there are benchmarks. If you remember from Chapter 3, we indicated that these are helpful because they are predictive of later student achievement. This allows teachers to determine who is on track and who needs additional assistance to be successful at reading. We provide benchmark scores in Table 4.2. The benchmark scores represent the lowest score we would accept that would indicate a student is *not* at risk for future academic failure.

Norms for Early Reading CBM

In addition to benchmarks, norms for LSF CBM are also available. The norms are helpful because they provide a way of comparing a student's score to the performance of others in his grade or at his instructional level. The benchmarks and norms can both be used to determine how much growth we would expect a student to make. Table 4.3 provides information on norms for LSF CBM for kindergarten and grade 1. There currently are no norms for WIF CBM.

TABLE 4.2. Benchmarks for LSF and WIF CBM

Grade	Task	Benchmark
Kindergarten	LSF	40 correct letter sounds per 1 minute
1	WIF	50 correct words from list per 1 minute

Note. Based on Fuchs and Fuchs (2004).

TABLE 4.3. Norms for LSF CBM: Letter Sounds Correct (LSC)

Grade	Percentile	AIMSweb (2008)[a] Fall (LSC)	Winter (LSC)	Spring (LSC)
Kindergarten	90%	21	43	53
	75%	11	32	43
	50%	**3**	**19**	**32**
	25%	0	8	20
	10%	—	2	11
1	90%	47	59	62
	75%	37	49	52
	50%	**27**	**38**	**41**
	25%	16	27	30
	10%	8	16	20

[a]2008 data updated for third printing.

HOW TO USE THE INFORMATION TO WRITE EARLY READING IEP GOALS AND OBJECTIVES

Using the same format presented in Chapter 3, here are some examples of using Early Reading CBM data to write goals and objectives. The principles are the same: time, learner, behavior (e.g., produces sounds, reads), level (kindergarten, first grade), content (e.g., reading), material (LSF/WIF CBM progress-monitoring material), and criteria (will reflect the norms or benchmarks for that skill including time and accuracy).

EXAMPLE OF GOALS

- LSF goal
  - In 30 weeks, Lindsay will produce letter sounds from a kindergarten reading sheet of random letters from LSF CBM progress-monitoring material at 35 LSC in 1 minute with greater than 95% accuracy.
- WIF goal
  - In 30 weeks, Tanasha will read aloud a first-grade reading list of high-frequency words from WIF CBM progress-monitoring material, at 50 WIC in 1 minute with greater than 95% accuracy.

The same principles apply to writing objectives, but one should use a shorter time frame.

EXAMPLE OF OBJECTIVES

- LSF objective
  - In 10 weeks, Lindsay will produce letter sounds from a kindergarten reading sheet of random letters from LSF CBM progress-monitoring material at 15 LSC in 1 minute with greater than 95% accuracy.

- WIF objective
  - In 10 weeks, Tanasha will read aloud a first-grade reading list of high-frequency words from WIF CBM progress-monitoring material at 25 WIC in 1 minute with greater than 95% accuracy.

FREQUENTLY ASKED QUESTIONS ABOUT EARLY READING CBM

1. *What happens if I start the stopwatch and the student starts reading silently?* You should stop the student. Get a different sheet at the same difficulty level, remind him that he needs to read aloud so that you can hear him, and start over, including reading the directions.

2. *If the student is not making good progress, should I lower the goal?* No. The first step should be to determine what skills the student is missing that is preventing him from making progress, teach those skills, and continue to monitor his progress. If you don't know what skills to teach, you may need to give a diagnostic evaluation, such as using Mastery Measurement.

3. *How long do I have to wait to raise the goal if the student is performing better than I thought he would?* After collecting at least six to eight data points, if the student has four *consecutive* data points above the goal line, then it should be raised.

4. *Can I make my own early reading sheets or do I have to purchase them?* We recommend that you purchase them to save time and to ensure that they are all of equivalent difficulty level, but you could make your own sheets.

5. *How much training does it typically take to learn how to do Early Reading CBM?* We have found that after practicing with seven to ten students, people are typically very good at conducting CBM.

6. *Can I change the directions or how I score the sheets/lists?* No. These measures were researched using the standardized procedures we have provided. If the directions or scoring criteria are changed, then the measure is changed, and we do not know what the reliability and validity are.

7. *Can I preteach the letter sounds or the words on the list?* No. This is an assessment and the goal is to determine what skills a student has without help. It is a good thing to teach letter sounds and words, but it is important not to combine the testing and teaching of these skills.

8. *How are CBM and DIBELS alike and different?* CBM and DIBELS are alike in that they use the same measurement techniques which include rate and accuracy. In fact, DIBELS measures were specifically modeled after CBM measures. CBM and DIBELS are different in that DIBELS includes early literacy assessments that measure phonemic awareness.

9. *Can I use benchmark scores on LSF and WIF CBM to put students in instructional groups?* Yes, if you have students with similar instructional needs. These groups should be flexible and students should be evaluated and regrouped every 6–8 weeks.

10. *Not everyone in my class is on the same instructional level. Should I still give them all the same LSF or WIF CBM sheets?* Yes. Because these skills are basic, all students in kindergarten should get LSF and all students in first grade should get WIF. If you have a student in first grade who is not successful on WIF, you could progress monitor him on LSF. The best way to handle this is to give both LSF and WIF each week so that you have an indication of how he is doing in both skills. Remember, when you screen/benchmark, it should always be done on students' grade-level skills (e.g., LSF for kindergarten and WIF for first grade).

11. *What should I do with the scored sheets?* This information can be kept in a portfolio along with the graphed data to demonstrate progress over the year.

12. *I only have 20 LSF or WIF CBM sheets, but I need to progress monitor for 35 weeks. Is it OK to use the same sheets again?* Yes. Once you have used all 20, start using them again. The student probably doesn't remember specific items he did 20 weeks ago. This also means that you should not use the sheets as homework or additional practice if you want to use them again.

RESOURCES AND FURTHER READING

Fuchs, L. S., Fuchs, D., & Compton, D. L. (2004). Monitoring early reading development in first grade: Word identification fluency versus nonsense word fluency. *Exceptional Children, 71*, 7–21.

Good, R. H., & Kaminski, R. A. (1996). Assessment for instructional decisions: Toward a proactive/prevention model of decision-making for early literacy skills. *School Psychology Quarterly, 11*, 326–336.

Good, R. H., Simmons, D. C., & Smith, S. B. (1998). Effective academic interventions in the United States: Evaluating and enhancing the acquisition of early reading skills. *School Psychology Review, 27*(1), 45–56.

Kaminski, R. A., & Good R. H. (1996). Toward a technology for assessing early literacy skills. *School Psychology Review, 25*, 215–227.

Speece, D. L., Mills, C., Ritchey, K. D., & Hillman, E. (2003). Initial evidence that letter fluency tasks are valid indicators of early reading skills. *The Journal of Special Education, 36*, 223–233.

INTERNET RESOURCES FOR EARLY READING

Florida Center for Reading Research
www.fcrr.org/assessment.htm

Intervention Central—CBM Warehouse
www.interventioncentral.org/htmdocs/interventions/cbmwarehouse.shtml

National Center on Student Progress Monitoring
www.studentprogress.org

Official DIBELS Homepage
www.dibels.uoregon.edu

Research Institute on Progress Monitoring
www.progressmonitoring.org

5

How to Conduct Spelling CBM

with TESSIE ROSE

OVERVIEW OF WHY TO CONDUCT SPELLING CBM

Spelling is an important skill for writing and evaluating that also provides information about a student's decoding. Good spellers are always good readers, but the reverse is not always true; a poor speller can be a good reader or a poor reader. Spelling CBM assesses students' ability to generalize learned spelling rules in novel tasks in addition to the number of words students can spell correctly.

Spelling CBM is a short, sensitive measure of spelling achievement. It can serve as an alternative to traditional weekly spelling tests, which often cannot distinguish between students' actual spelling skill and their ability to memorize or copy words (Loeffler, 2005). It has been field tested for more than 25 years and has been used successfully with general education students (Fuchs et al., 1993) and students with disabilities (Fuchs, Fuchs, & Hamlett, 1989). As with all other CBM tasks, the information obtained provides a database for each student so that appropriate instructional decisions can be made in a timely manner.

MATERIALS NEEDED TO CONDUCT SPELLING CBM

The first step in administering Spelling CBM is to acquire the appropriate materials:

1. Different but equivalent grade-level spelling lists.
2. Directions for administering and scoring Spelling CBM.

Tessie Rose is currently an assistant professor of special education at the University of Nevada–Las Vegas. She received her PhD at the University of Utah in special education with an emphasis in curriculum and assessment.

3. Lined paper and writing utensils for student responses.
4. A stopwatch or countdown timer that displays seconds.
5. A quiet testing environment to work with students.
6. An equal-interval graph or a graphing program to plot the data.

Spelling CBM Lists

The spelling lists should have different words, include the same number of total letters, be equivalent in grade level, and include 12 words for first and second grade and 17 words for third grade and above. The lists are skills-based measures, meaning that they are composed of items/words selected from across the whole year's spelling curriculum. There are some programs that have already created grade-level spelling lists with equal numbers of correct letter sequences (which makes scoring much faster). These commercial programs typically provide 20–40 alternate forms representing the year-long curriculum. A source for obtaining spelling lists is provided in Box 5.1.

Purchasing premade lists may not be an option in some situations, but teachers can create their own grade-level spelling lists. Lists must be similar in the number of words and correct letter sequences (CLS). The words should be sampled equally from spelling lists found throughout the year-long curriculum. To obtain similar levels of CLS, choose the same number of three-, four-, five-, etc. -letter words for each list. Although specific CLS data do not exist for each grade level, the following can be used as guidelines: first- and second-grade lists should have 55–70 CLS and upper-level lists should have 125–155 CLS.

Just like the other CBM measures, the first time Spelling CBM is administered three equivalent spelling lists should be used, whether you are going to be conducting screening/benchmarking or progress monitoring. This should be conducted in one testing ses-

---

BOX 5.1. Where to Find Premade Spelling CBM Lists

$ indicates there is a cost for the lists and/or graphing program.
⌨ indicates computerized administration available.
✍ indicates data management and graphing available.

AIMSweb (Pearson) $✍

Website: *www.aimsweb.com*
Phone: 866-323-6194
Address: Harcourt Assessment, Inc.
AIMSweb Customer Service
P.O. Box 599700
San Antonio, TX 78259
Products: • Spelling (30 progress monitoring lists, 3 benchmarking lists for grades 1–8)

sion, but it can occur across consecutive days if needed. We recommend doing it in one session to save set-up time and obtain a more accurate score. The median score of these three samples will be used to provide the first data point on the student's graph. After that, 20–30 different but equivalent lists will be used to monitor student progress in spelling throughout the year.

Spelling CBM can be administered individually or to a group. The spelling lists will be needed along with the directions and a timer. The student(s) should have lined paper and a pencil or pen. It may be helpful to give each student a spiral notebook for his responses. This allows teachers and students to see progress over time as well as provide a record of student responses. It is also helpful in situations where the measure is given to all students each week even though just a few are being progress monitored. See Figures 5.1 and 5.2 for examples of a spelling list and a scored spelling list.

AIMSweb® Standard Spelling Progress Monitor Assessment List #4 (3rd Grade)

Given By: _____   Date Given: __ / __ / __

ID	Word	CLS	CCLS
1	tape	5	5
2	supplier	9	14
3	jelly	6	20
4	rooster	8	28
5	cricket	8	36
6	sheriff	8	44
7	house	6	50
8	waste Don't waste good food.	6	56
9	wear What are you going to wear?	5	61
10	away	5	66
11	led She led the class.	4	70
12	ear	4	74
13	woolen	7	81
14	obeyed	7	88
15	onto	5	93
16	wagging	8	101
17	watermelon	11	112
	Total CLS	**112**	

Note. CCLS = Cumulative CLS.

FIGURE 5.1. Example of teacher/examiner Spelling CBM list. Reprinted from AIMSweb (2003). Copyright 2003 by Edformation, Inc. Reprinted by permission.

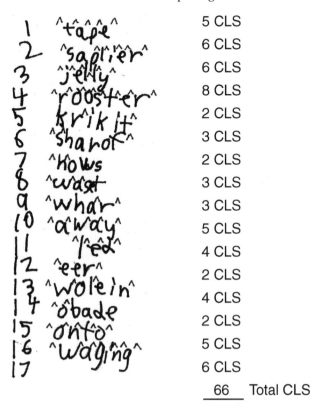

1	^tape^	5 CLS
2	^saplier^	6 CLS
3	jelly^	6 CLS
4	^rooster^	8 CLS
5	krik it^	2 CLS
6	^sharot^	3 CLS
7	^kows	2 CLS
8	^wast	3 CLS
9	^whar^	3 CLS
10	^away^	5 CLS
11	^red^	4 CLS
12	^eer^	2 CLS
13	^wolein^	4 CLS
14	^obade	2 CLS
15	^onto^	5 CLS
16	^waging^	6 CLS
17		

66 Total CLS

FIGURE 5.2. Example of student Spelling CBM list scored.

DIRECTIONS AND SCORING PROCEDURES FOR SPELLING CBM

For your convenience, Appendix B includes a reproducible version of the directions and scoring rules for Spelling CBM.

Directions for Spelling CBM[1]

1. Select an appropriate grade-level spelling list.
2. Have students number their papers 1 to 12 for first and second graders or 1 to 17 for third grade and up.
3. Say: *"I am going to read some words to you. I want you to write the words on the sheet in front of you. Write the first word on the first line, the second word on the second line, and so on. I'll give you 10 seconds [7 seconds for grade 3 and up] to spell each word. When I say the next word, try to write it, even if you haven't finished the last one. Are there any questions?"*

---

[1]Adapted from Shinn (1989).

4. Say the first word and trigger stopwatch or timer for 2 minutes.
5. Say each word twice. Use homonyms in a sentence.
6. Say a new word every 10 seconds (grades 1 and 2) or 7 seconds (grade 3 and up).
7. At the end of 2 minutes, say: ***"Thank you. Put your pencils down."***

Scoring Spelling CBM

Spelling CBM can be scored for correct letter sequences (CLS) and words spelled correctly (WSC). CLS is the total number of pairs of letters that are in the correct sequence; WSC is the total number of words spelled correctly.

1. Count the total number of correct letter sequences to obtain the CLS score.
2. Count the total number of words spelled correctly to obtain the WSC score.

CLS requires more time to score but also offers a more sensitive measure to gauge student improvement. CLS can provide diagnostic information, assess the effectiveness of spelling instruction, and monitor students' progress. A correct letter sequence includes the beginning space to the first letter, letter to letter, a letter to punctuation, punctuation to a letter, and an end letter to a space. CLS is scored using an upper caret (^) to identify each correct sequence. Nothing is used to identify incorrect letter sequences. The CLS for each word is equal to the number of letters in the word plus one, except when punctuation is used; then it is the number of letters in the word plus two.

WSC is easier to score. Each correctly spelled word or its corresponding number is circled and the total number of circled words is the WSC. WSC is currently used in many spelling programs as an indicator of general spelling skill.

Comparison between WSC and CLS

Example: Five dictated words, scoring for WSC and CLS, and possible CLS

Dictated Words	Student Response	WSC	CLS	Possible CLS
heel	1. ^h^el^	0	3	5 ^h^e^e^l^
wise	2. ^w^ize^	0	3	5 ^w^i^s^e^
don't	3. ^d^o^nt^	0	4	6 ^d^o^n^'^t^
speak	4. ^s^p^e^a^k^	1	6	6 ^s^p^e^a^k^
dinner	5. ^d^i^n^n^e^r^	1	7	7 ^d^i^n^n^e^r^

This example demonstrates how CLS is more sensitive to student improvement than WSC is. For WSC, the student got 2 of 5 words correct, which is 40% correct. For CLS, the student got 23 of 29 letter sequences correct, which is 79% correct.

With WSC, the student gets the same credit (0) when spelling *heel* if he writes "xxzz" or "hel." Obviously one is closer to correct than the other. Using CLS gives the teacher, student, and parent a better idea of *how* close the student is to learning spelling patterns and getting the answer correct.

Scoring Correct Letter Sequences

- CLS is the number of correct sequences related to spelling, the space before and after the word, and the letter to punctuation (before and after). When scoring CLS, the scorer places a caret (^) to indicate each correct sequence.
  Example: Dictated word *chair*
  - ^c^h^a^i^r^ = 6 CLS
  - ^c^h^a r s = 3 CLS
- Compound words: Words need to stay together without a space.
  Example: Dictated word *downhill*
  - ^d^o^w^n^h^i^l^l^ = 9 CLS
  - ^d^o^w^n h^i^l^l^ = 8 CLS
- Apostrophe: The spaces before and after an apostrophe are counted.
  Example: Dictated word *o'clock*
  - ^o^'^c^l^o^c^k^ = 8 CLS
  - ^o c^l^o^c^k^ = 6 CLS
- Hyphens: The spaces before and after a hyphen are counted.
  Example: Dictated word *sister-in-law*
  - ^s^i^s^t^e^r^-^i^n^-^l^a^w^ = 14 CLS
  - ^s^i^s^t^e^r i^n l^a^w^ = 10 CLS
- Capitalization: A word that should be capitalized must begin with a capital letter.
  Example: Dictated word *April*
  - ^A^p^r^i^l^ = 6 CLS
  - a p^r^i^l^ = 4 CLS
- Repeated letters in sequence: Words with letters that are repeated in sequence are scored the same as if each letter were different.
  Example: Dictated word *bloom*
  - ^b^l^o^o^m^ = 6 CLS
  - ^b^l^o m^ = 4 CLS
    or
  - ^b^l o^m^ = 4 CLS
- Additional letters: Additional letters are not counted twice.
  Example: Dictated word *correct*
  - ^c^o^r^r^e^c^t^ = 8 CLS
  - ^c^o^r r r^e^c^t^ = 7 CLS
- Insertions: Extra letters at the beginning and end are not counted.
  Example: Dictated word *phone*
  - ^p^h^o^n^e^ = 6 CLS
  - fp^h^o^n^e^ = 5 CLS
  - ^p^h^o^n^e y = 5 CLS

Special Administration and Scoring Considerations for Spelling CBM

1. It is vital that each word is pronounced clearly and at an audible level.
2. Use a prompt for younger students to keep them on the right number every four to five words. Say, for example, "**Number 5 is . . .** (*insert word*)."
3. Students should not receive additional instructions or corrections during any part of the test administration.

HOW OFTEN SHOULD SPELLING CBM BE GIVEN?

In Chapter 3, we provide additional details on how often and when to administer CBM for the different purposes of screening/benchmarking, progress monitoring, and survey-level assessment. Below we provide only an outline for screening/benchmarking and progress monitoring as criteria for survey-level assessment to determine instructional levels have not yet been developed for Spelling CBM. We suggest you refer to Chapter 3 for a more in-depth discussion on how often and when to give CBM for these different purposes.

- Screening/benchmarking = all students in a classroom or grade level, once per quarter (three to four times per school year); typically conducted in the fall, winter, and spring.
- Progress monitoring = students in the bottom 25% of the class based on the screening/benchmarking assessment, at least one time per week; preferably two times per week. This includes any student who is considered at risk based on norms or benchmark criteria.
- Monthly progress monitoring of CLS and WSC is suggested for all students; these data provide teachers with more information about the typical progress of students and the effectiveness of classroom instruction.

HOW MUCH TIME DOES IT TAKE TO ADMINISTER AND SCORE SPELLING CBM?

The time needed to score each student list will depend on the proficiency of the speller, the grade level, and the experience of the scorer. Whether you are giving a test to a class of 25 or an individual student, the time is still 2 minutes for the test itself plus your time to get the student(s) ready and for you to collect the sheets. We would estimate that once the students are familiar with the process, it should take from 5 to 10 minutes to administer the test.

Knowing the number of CLS for each word and for the total list will assist in scoring. First, it will not be necessary to count the CLS for each word if they are all spelled correctly. Second, if the student misses only a few CLS, you can subtract the difference from the total CLS as opposed to adding the CLS for each word. Third, it may be easier to use a felt tip pen and make dots instead of carets; however, this should only be used after you have become proficient at scoring Spelling CBM. We estimate that it would take no longer than 10–15 seconds to score WSC and 30 seconds to score CLS if the total CLS is already known.

EXPECTED GROWTH RATES AND NORMS FOR SPELLING CBM

As mentioned in previous chapters, it is just as important to know how much growth we can expect a student to make as it is to know where she is starting. We use the baseline score (the median of the three Spelling CBM tests) to tell us where the student is starting and the growth, benchmarks, and norms to tell us what kind of progress we should aim for.

When a student's behavior (i.e., actual progress) does not meet the expected growth rate, it is our obligation to find a way to fix that problem. Teachers might do this by building up a weak subskill, increasing the length of daily lessons, or altering the way they respond when an error is made, but not by lowering expectations. Learning is the result of instruction. When the rate of learning is inadequate, it doesn't always mean there is something wrong with the student. It does mean the instruction needs to be changed.

How Much Progress Can We Expect in Spelling?

Growth rates for progress in CLS were investigated by Fuchs and colleagues (1993) and are presented in Table 5.1. There currently are no growth rates established for WSC. The typical weekly rates of improvement should not be viewed as the maximum progress possible. Progress levels beyond these are possible and will, in fact, be needed to bring students who have fallen behind up to the levels of their peers.

Weekly spelling growth rates for first-grade students are not found in the literature, but students typically make the most progress in spelling during their first couple of years in school. Therefore, it can be assumed that first-grade students will make progress

TABLE 5.1. Weekly Growth
Rates on Spelling CBM:
Correct Letter Sequences (CLS)

Grade	Growth rates per week (CLS)
2	1–1.5
3	0.65–1
4	0.45–0.85
5	0.3–0.65
6	0.3–0.65

Note. Data from Fuchs et al. (1993).

similar to if not greater than second-grade students. Students monitored on seventh- and eighth-grade spelling lists can expect similar or slightly lower growth rates than students in fifth and sixth grade.

Norms for Spelling CBM

Norms can be used to compare a student's score to the performance of others in her grade. The norms can be used to gauge a student's level of performance and rate of progress over time.

Norms for CLS are presented in Table 5.2.

HOW TO USE THE INFORMATION
TO WRITE SPELLING IEP GOALS AND OBJECTIVES

Using the same format presented in Chapter 3, here are some examples of using Spelling CBM data to write goals and objectives. The principles are the same: time, learner, behavior (e.g., spells), level (e.g., grade), content (e.g., spelling), material (Spelling CBM progress-monitoring material), and criteria (will reflect the norms or benchmarks for that skill including time and accuracy).

EXAMPLE OF GOALS

- Spelling goal
  - In 30 weeks, Roberto will spell words from a fourth-grade spelling list from Spelling CBM progress-monitoring material at 70 CLS in 2 minutes with greater than 95% accuracy.

The same principles apply to writing objectives, but one should use a shorter time frame.

EXAMPLE OF OBJECTIVES

- Spelling objective
  - In 10 weeks, Roberto will spell words from a fourth-grade spelling list from Spelling CBM progress-monitoring material at 25 CLS in 2 minutes with greater than 95% accuracy.

FREQUENTLY ASKED QUESTIONS ABOUT SPELLING CBM

1. *Can I give students the list prior to the assessment?* No. This assessment is a general measure of students' skill at applying the spelling rules they have been previously taught. Giving students the list prior to the assessment increases the chance that students will attempt to memorize the words instead of learning the spelling skills being taught.

TABLE 5.2. Norms for Spelling CBM: Correct Letter Sequences (CLS)

Grade	Percentile	AIMSweb (2008)[a]		
		Fall (CLS)	Winter (CLS)	Spring (CLS)
1	90%	43	51	55
	75%	36	46	51
	50%	**28**	**41**	**45**
	25%	16	36	38
	10%	5	26	30
2	90%	64	66	68
	75%	58	62	65
	50%	**49**	**55**	**61**
	25%	39	45	55
	10%	28	34	46
3	90%	103	107	111
	75%	94	101	108
	50%	**80**	**90**	**100**
	25%	61	76	86
	10%	44	58	65
4	90%	115	124	122
	75%	107	118	117
	50%	**92**	**107**	**107**
	25%	71	89	91
	10%	52	67	68
5	90%	136	133	134
	75%	130	127	129
	50%	**115**	**116**	**120**
	25%	90	97	103
	10%	64	70	77
6	90%	142	141	147
	75%	135	133	140
	50%	**120**	**119**	**129**
	25%	99	102	110
	10%	70	82	85
7	90%	136	145	144
	75%	127	135	137
	50%	**112**	**121**	**124**
	25%	91	100	96
	10%	62	77	70
8	90%	145	142	144
	75%	139	135	132
	50%	**129**	**122**	**118**
	25%	107	102	94
	10%	42	73	64

[a]2008 data updated for third printing.

2. *The list for this week doesn't include the spelling rules I just taught. Can I choose one that does?* No. Avoid teaching to the test and remember Spelling CBM is designed to assess general, not specific, skill mastery.

3. *What if a student becomes distracted or fails to participate during the classroom administration?* Complete the classroom administration and then individually administer a different list at a later time.

4. *Not everyone in my class is on the same instructional level. Should I still give them all the same spelling list?* All students should be screened/benchmarked on their grade level, but they should be progress monitored on their instructional level, especially if they are receiving instruction on that level. The best way to handle this is to give both the grade-level and the instructional-level spelling lists each week so that you have an indication of how they are doing given the instruction they are receiving (instructional level) and how well it is transferring to more difficult words (grade level).

5. *What if an interruption occurs during administration (e.g., fire alarm, school bell, class visitor, etc.)?* If a significant interruption occurs, stop administering the spelling list and administer a different list at a more appropriate time.

6. *Should I teach students the spelling rules they miss on the spelling lists?* Yes. Whenever students are missing previously taught rules, it is beneficial to reteach the material. This may be an indication that students did not fully understand the concept. Teachers should, however, continue to use the scope and sequence presented in the curriculum.

7. *What if I cannot tell what letter the student wrote?* In cases of doubt, do not give the student credit and be sure to tell her why. In extreme cases, administer another spelling list and ask the student to use her best handwriting.

8. *Can I use Spelling CBM for my students' weekly spelling test grade?* Yes. If your spelling curriculum matches the Spelling CBM lists (e.g., affixes, long vowels, compound words), it can be used for your weekly spelling test grade. You would want to make sure that the students and parents understand what the score means as well as what the goal for the year is.

9. *Can I use the norms to put students in instructional groups?* It is not recommended. Other assessment tools (e.g., Words Their Way Spelling Inventory) are more appropriate for identifying skill strengths and weaknesses in spelling. Instructional groupings will be more successful if they are based on student needs that can be used to guide instruction.

10. *If the student is not making progress, should I lower the goal?* No. Instead, assess the student's needs and provide additional interventions to address the target areas.

11. *What should I do with the scored spelling sheets?* This information can be kept in a portfolio along with the graphed data to demonstrate progress over the year.

12. *I only have 20 Spelling CBM lists, but I need to progress monitor for 35 weeks. Is it OK to use the same lists again?* Yes. Once you have used all 20, start using them again. The student probably doesn't remember specific items she did 20 weeks ago. This also means that you should not use the lists as homework or additional practice if you want to use them again.

RESOURCES AND FURTHER READING

Fuchs, L. S., Allinder, R. M., & Hamlett, C. L. (1990). An analysis of spelling curricula and teachers' skills at identifying error types. *Remedial and Special Education, 11*(1), 42–52.

Fuchs, L. S., Fuchs, D., Hamlett, C. L., & Allinder, R. M. (1991). The contribution of skills analysis to curriculum-based measurement in spelling. *Exceptional Children, 57,* 443–452.

Shinn, M. R., & Shinn, M. M. (2002). *AIMSweb training workbook: Administration and scoring of spelling curriculum-based measurement (S-CBM) for use in general outcome measurement.* Eden Prairie, MN: Edformation.

6

How to Conduct Writing CBM

with TESSIE ROSE

OVERVIEW OF WHY TO CONDUCT WRITING CBM

Writing is a critical skill that students need to master in order to succeed in school and life. Fortunately, there are specific skills that provide good indications of students' overall writing skills, allowing one to determine what writing skills they mastered as well as to monitor their progress. As with all other CBM tasks, this information provides a database for each student so that appropriate instructional decisions can be made in a timely manner. We know that monitoring students' progress and making instructional decisions based on their progress leads to better outcomes for students. So what is Writing CBM?

Writing CBM is a short, simple measure of students' writing skill. Students are required to write for 3 minutes on an instructional-level story starter and are scored on specific writing skills. Howell and Nolet (2000) identified several components of written communication pertinent to student progress in written language. They included writing fluency, syntactic maturity, vocabulary or semantic maturity, content, and conventions (e.g., spelling, punctuation, and capitalization). Numerous studies have presented curriculum-based measures available for many of these target areas, including total words written (TWW), words spelled correctly (WSC), correct writing sequences (CWS), and total correct punctuation (TCP) (Gansle, Noell, VanDerHeyden, Naquin, & Slider, 2002; Videen, Deno, & Martson, 1982). Writing CBM has been used successfully with secondary students (Espin, Scierka, Skare, & Halverson, 1999), middle school students (Espin et al., 2000), elementary students (Deno, Mirkin, Lowry, & Kuehnle, 1980; Deno, Marston, & Mirkin, 1982; Videen et al., 1982), and students with learning disabilities (Watkinson & Lee, 1992).

MATERIALS NEEDED TO CONDUCT WRITING CBM

1. Different but equivalent story starters that are grade appropriate.
2. Directions for administering and scoring Writing CBM.
3. Lined paper and writing utensils for student responses.
4. A stopwatch or countdown timer that displays seconds.
5. A quiet testing environment to work with students.
6. An equal-interval graph or a graphing program to plot the data.

Writing CBM Story Starters

The story starters should be equivalent in grade level and should be of the same interest for that grade. Story starters are short oral or written sentences that begin the writing process. They are designed to elicit more than a yes/no or short-answer response. The story starters should also elicit the writing skills the students are expected to master throughout the school year. While the story starters should be different, they should all be of equivalent difficulty (i.e., at the same grade level). The best way to assure this is to purchase generic story starters that have been developed specifically for this purpose. A source for obtaining story starters is provided in Box 6.1. In addition, we have included some story starters that we have used in Figure 6.1.

Just like the other CBM measures, the first time Writing CBM is administered three equivalent story starters should be used, whether you are going to be conducting screening/benchmarking or progress monitoring. This should be conducted in one testing session, but it can occur across consecutive days if needed. We recommend doing it in one session to save set-up time and obtain a more accurate score. The median score of these three samples will be used to provide the first data point on the student's graph. After that, 20–30 different but equivalent story starters will be used to monitor student progress in writing throughout the year.

BOX 6.1. Where to Find Premade Writing CBM Story Starters

$ indicates there is a cost for the story starters and/or graphing program.

💻 indicates computerized administration available.

✍ indicates data management and graphing available.

AIMSweb (Pearson) $✍

Website: *www.aimsweb.com*

Phone: 866-323-6194

Address: Harcourt Assessment, Inc.
AIMSweb Customer Service
P.O. Box 599700
San Antonio, TX 78259

Products: • Writing story starters (125 across grades 1–8)

Primary

- The funniest thing I did this summer was . . .
- The best part about school is . . .
- Today I woke up and . . .
- Yesterday I made a beautiful . . .
- The scariest Halloween I had was . . .
- The best vacation I ever took was . . .
- The dog was barking so loud that . . .
- Yesterday the class went to the zoo and . . .
- I was walking home from school one day when . . .
- I was walking to school one day when . . .
- My favorite game to play during recess is . . .
- If I could fly I would go . . .
- A little worm was crawling down the sidewalk when he . . .
- The dog climbed on the table and . . .
- There are many fun things to do at the park like . . .
- The best vacation I ever had was . . . .
- I could not find my puppy anywhere. I . . .
- I could not find my kitty anywhere. I . . .
- My dog saw a cat. I called out . . .
- At the circus I saw an elephant that was . . .
- When I was flying on a magic carpet . . .
- My favorite toy is . . .
- He knew something was different when . . .
- I looked out my window and to my surprise . . .
- On my way home from school I found a . . .

Intermediate

- I had never been afraid of being home alone at night until . . .
- "What is it?" I whispered to my friend, when suddenly . . .
- The lights went out and . . .
- I couldn't believe I had been voted class president! My first item of business was . . .
- When the alarm sounded I . . .
- I opened the front door and found a huge package and . . .
- One morning I woke up and sitting at the end of my bed was . . .
- As soon as I saw the large dog I knew . . .
- The dancer came onto the stage and . . .
- My day was going bad until . . .
- One day in the cafeteria, I saw some food on the ground . . .
- The dog looked sick and I heard sirens but saw no one . . .
- I looked out the window and to my surprise the world was white. Everything was covered with a blanket of snow. I . . .
- I saw the lighting and then I heard the thunder. I thought . . .
- Instead of going to bed last night, I decided to . . .
- While I was in my bed sleeping last night, I was awoken by . . .
- He knew something was different when . . .
- I was walking to school when . . .
- Out of a hole in the ground arose a great big . . .
- As I was walking through the cemetery I could hear . . .

(continued)

FIGURE 6.1. Example of story starters for Writing CBM.

Advanced

- It was like a dream come true when I . . .
- I knew I was in trouble when I couldn't find . . .
- "I knew it was you," I shouted when I noticed that . . .
- Once the noise stopped, everyone began to look around for what it was. It seemed to be . . .
- We arrived at the hotel expecting to be greeted, but instead . . .
- Number seven was winding up for the pitch when all of a sudden . . .
- Joe and Bob slowly crept up the creaky stairs and knocked on the door of the old house when . . .
- The teenagers were hiking through the forest when they came across an old rundown cabin that was . . .
- The light shined faintly through the fog, making it difficult to . . .
- The clerk at the store was annoyed, because . . .
- My dog was running toward the President and was about to . . .
- I could not sleep last night because . . .
- The funniest trick I ever played on _____ was . . .
- The waves were enormous and wind furious when all of a sudden . . .
- When I was swimming in the lake, I noticed . . .
- As I was coming out of the long tunnel, I happened to see . . .
- Mrs. Smith doesn't understand. I was only trying to . . .

FIGURE 6.1. *(continued)*

Writing CBM can be administered individually or to a group. The story starters will be needed along with the directions and a timer. The student(s) should have lined paper and a pencil or pen. It may be helpful to give each student a spiral notebook for student responses. This allows teachers and students to see progress over time as well as provide a record of student responses. It is also helpful in situations where the measure is given to all students each week even though just a few are being progress monitored. See Figure 6.2 for an example of a student's response to the story starter. "The best birthday I ever had was . . . ."

FIGURE 6.2. Example of student Writing CBM.

DIRECTIONS AND SCORING PROCEDURES FOR WRITING CBM

For your convenience, Appendix B includes a reproducible version of the directions and scoring rules for Writing CBM.

Directions for Writing CBM[1]

1. Provide students with a pencil and piece of lined paper or writing notebook.
2. Select an appropriate story starter.
3. Say: *"Today I want you to write a story. I am going to read a sentence to you first and then I want you to compose a short story about what happens. You will have 1 minute to think about what you will write and 3 minutes to write your story. Remember to do your best work. If you do not know how to spell a word, you should guess. Are there any questions?* (Pause) *Put your pencils down and listen. For the next minute, think about* . . . (insert story starter)."
4. After reading the story starter, begin your stopwatch and allow **1 minute** for the student(s) to think. (Monitor students so that they do not begin writing.) After **30 seconds** say: *"You should be thinking about* . . . (insert story starter)." At the end of **1 minute**, restart your stopwatch for 3 minutes and say: *"Now begin writing."*
5. Monitor students' attention to the task. Encourage the students to work if they are not writing.
6. After **90 seconds** say: *"You should be writing about* . . . (insert story starter)."
7. At the end of **3 minutes** say: *"Thank you. Put your pencils down."*

Scoring Writing CBM

1. Count the total number of words written to obtain the total words written (TWW) score.
2. Count the total number of words spelled correctly to obtain the words spelled correctly (WSC) score.
3. Count the total number of correct writing sequences to obtain the correct writing sequence (CWS) score.

While these are the most common procedures for scoring Writing CBM, there are other procedures that have been used to score student responses. For example, Espin and colleagues (1999) used the number of long words or characters per word. Other potential scoring procedures include the number of different words, number of nouns, number of verbs, number of adjectives, total punctuation marks, correct punctuation marks, correct capital letters, complete sentences, words in complete sentences, sentence fragments, and simple sentences. Additional research is needed to confirm the validity of these measures (Gansle et al., 2002; Tindal & Parker, 1991). Therefore, this chapter will

---

[1]Adapted from AIMSweb (Powell-Smith & Shinn, 2004).

only include scoring procedures for TWW, WSC, and CWS. Figure 6.3 is an example of a scored student passage using these three scoring procedures.

Scoring Total Words Written

- Total words written (TWW) is the number of words written regardless of spelling or context. When scoring TWW, the scorer <u>underlines each word written</u> and records the total number of words written (see Figure 6.3). Words are defined as any letter or group of letters, including misspelled or nonsense words, that have a space before and after them.
  - <u>I read the book</u>.   TWW = 4
  - <u>I red the book</u>.   TWW = 4
  - <u>I wont to go</u>.   TWW = 4
  - <u>I wanna go</u>.   TWW = 3
  - <u>Iv grqx zznip</u>.   TWW = 3
- Abbreviations: Common abbreviations are counted as words (e.g., Dr., Mrs., TV).
  - <u>Dr. Smith came in</u>.   TWW = 4
  - <u>I like TV</u>.   TWW = 3
- Hyphenated words: Each morpheme in a hyphenated word separated by a hyphen is counted as an individual word if it can stand alone. Prefixes separated by a hyphen are not counted as words, although the root word is counted.
  - <u>My sister-in-law came to visit</u>.   TWW = 7
  - <u>It is cold-blooded</u>.   TWW = 4

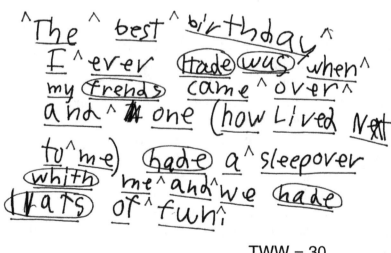

TWW = 30
WSC = 23
CWS = 15

FIGURE 6.3. Example of student Writing CBM scored.

○ I love to bar-b-que.   TWW = 4
○ We need to re-evaluate the cost. TWW = 6
- Titles and endings: Story titles and endings are counted as words written.
    ○ My Bad Day by Sarah   TWW = 5
    ○ The end   TWW = 2
- Numerals: Numerals, with the exception of dates and currency, are not counted as words unless they are written out (i.e., as words).
    ○ I have 3 cats.   TWW = 3
    ○ I have three cats.   TWW = 4
    ○ Today is August 13, 1974.   TWW = 5
    ○ I have $50.   TWW = 3
    ○ I have 50.   TWW = 2
    ○ I have 50 dollars.   TWW = 4
- Unusual characters: Unusual characters are not counted as words even if they are meant to take the place of a word.
    ○ Mary & I went home.   TWW = 4
    ○ She won a lot of $.   TWW = 5
    ○ I will give you 50%.   TWW = 4

Scoring Words Spelled Correctly

WSC is the number of correctly spelled words, regardless of context. Words are counted in WSC if they can be found in the English language. Incorrectly spelled words should be circled (see Figure 6.3). WSC is calculated by subtracting the total number of circled words from the TWW. As with TWW, additional scoring rules apply to WSC.

- Abbreviations: Abbreviations must be spelled correctly.
    ○ I live on President Blvd.   WSC = 5
    ○ I live on President Bld.   WSC = 4
- Hyphenated words: Each morpheme counted as an individual word must be spelled correctly. If the morpheme cannot stand alone (e.g., prefix) and part of the word is incorrect, the entire word is counted as an incorrect spelling.
    ○ She is my sister-in-law.   WSC = 6
    ○ She is my sista-in-law.   WSC = 5
    ○ I need to re-evaluate this.   WSC = 5
    ○ I need to re-eveluate this.   WSC = 4
- Titles and endings: Words in the title or ending are counted in the words spelled correctly.
    ○ My Terrible Day   WSC = 3
    ○ My Terrable Day   WSC = 2
- Capitalization: Proper nouns must be capitalized unless the name is also a common noun. Capitalization of the first word in the sentence is not a requirement for the

word to be spelled correctly. Words are counted as spelled correctly even if they are capitalized incorrectly within the sentence.

- She sat with Bill.   WSC = 4
- she sat with Bill.   WSC = 4
- She sat with bill.   WSC = 4
- She sat with the bill.   WSC = 5
- She sat With the bill.   WSC = 5

- Reversed letters: Words containing letter reversals are not counted as errors unless the reversal causes the word to be spelled incorrectly. This typically applies with reversals of the following letters: *p, q, g, d, b, n, u.*
  - The pig was at the farm.   WSC = 6
  - The (qig) was at the farm.   WSC = 5
  - The big pig ate.   WSC = 4
  - The dig pig ate.   WSC = 4

- Contractions: In order for a contraction to be counted as correct, it must have the apostrophe in the correct place unless the word can stand alone.
  - Its my turn.   WSC = 3
  - It's my turn.   WSC = 3
  - She isn't here.   WSC = 3
  - She (isnt) here.   WSC = 2

Correct Writing Sequences

A CWS is "two adjacent, correctly spelled words that are acceptable within the context of the [written] phrase to a native speaker of the English language" (Videen et al., 1982, p. 7). It takes into account punctuation, syntax, semantics, spelling, and capitalization. When scoring CWS, a caret (^) is used to mark each correct word sequence. A space is implied at the beginning of a sentence. The following should be taken into consideration when scoring CWS.

- Spelling: Words must be spelled correctly to be counted in CWS. Words that are not counted in WSC or are circled words are *not* counted as correct word sequences.
  - ^ She ^ waited ^ for ^ me ^ at ^ the ^ store ^ .   CWS = 8
  - ^ She (waeted) for ^ me ^ at ^ the (stor.)   CWS = 4
- Capitalization: Capitalization at the beginning of the sentence is necessary. Proper nouns must be capitalized unless they can serve as common nouns in the given context. Incorrectly capitalized words are marked as incorrect CWS.
  - ^ She ^ is ^ coming ^ over ^ .   CWS = 5
  - she is ^ coming ^ over ^ .   CWS = 3
  - ^ She ^ sat ^ with bill.   CWS = 3
  - ^ She ^ sat ^ with ^ the ^ bill ^ . CWS = 6
  - ^ He ^ is ^ on ^ my Pillow.   CWS = 4

- Punctuation: Correct punctuation must be at the end of the sentence. Commas are not typically counted unless they are used in a series. In a series, they must be used correctly to be scored. Other punctuation marks are typically not counted as CWS.
  - ^ Mary ^ asked ^ if ^ I ^ would ^ come ^ over ^ . ^ I ^ said ^ no ^ .   CWS = 12
  - ^ Mary ^ asked ^ if ^ I ^ would ^ come ^ over i ^ said ^ no   CWS = 9
  - ^ I ^ have ^ a ^ cat, ^ dog ^ and ^ bird ^ .   CWS = 8
  - ^ I ^ have ^ a ^ cat dog ^ and ^ bird ^ .   CWS = 7
- Syntax: Words must be syntactically correct to be counted as CWS. Sentences that begin with a conjunction are considered to be syntactically correct.
  - ^ He ^ had ^ never ^ seen ^ the ^ movie ^ before ^ .   CWS = 8
  - ^ He ^ never seen ^ the ^ movie ever ^ .   CWS = 5
  - ^ And ^ he ^ wanted ^ to ^ go ^ see ^ it ^ with ^ me ^ .   CWS = 10
- Semantics: Words must be semantically correct to be counted in CWS.
  - ^ That ^ pig ^ is ^ too ^ fat ^ .   CWS = 6
  - ^ That ^ pig ^ is to fat ^ .   CWS = 4
- Story titles and endings: Story titles and endings are included in the scoring of CWS and must meet scoring criteria for spelling, punctuation, capitalization, syntax, and semantics to be counted in CWS.
  - ^ The ^ Big ^ Fat ^ Wedding ^ by ^ Billy ^   CWS = 7
  - ^ The ^ Big fat Wedding ^ by billy   CWS = 3
  - the big fat wedding   CWS = 0
  - ^ The ^ End ^ .   CWS = 3
  - ^ The end ^ .   CWS = 2

Special Administration and Scoring Considerations for Writing CBM

1. Although TWW and WSC are easy to score, they tend to yield fluency information only. The extra time needed to score CWS is suggested at all levels for students below grade level in writing. CWS scoring supplies a great deal of useful information about error patterns and missing skills. It is also more sensitive to instruction, so it makes a better tool for progress monitoring.

2. Directions should be read as presented above, and students should not receive additional instructions or corrections during any part of the test administration.

3. Test administrators may find that 3-minute written responses do not yield enough information, particularly for students struggling with writing. Longer samples using 5 and 10 minutes can be used for analysis, but the scores cannot be used in comparison to the norm if the normative sample used 3 minutes. Another option is to note where the student is at the end of 3 minutes to compare to the normative sample but then let him keep writing for an additional 2–7 minutes.

HOW OFTEN SHOULD WRITING CBM BE GIVEN?

In Chapter 3, we provide additional details on how often and when to administer CBM for the different purposes of screening/benchmarking, progress monitoring, and survey-level assessment. Below we provide only an outline for screening/benchmarking and progress monitoring as criteria for survey-level assessment to determine instructional levels have not yet been developed for Writing CBM. We suggest you refer to Chapter 3 for a more in-depth discussion on how often and when to give CBM for these different purposes.

- Screening/benchmarking = all students in a classroom or grade level, once per quarter (three to four times per school year); typically conducted in the fall, winter, and spring.
- Progress monitoring = students in the bottom 25% of the class based on the screening/benchmarking assessment, at least one time per week; preferably two times per week. This includes any student who is considered at risk based on norms.
- Monthly progress monitoring of all students can provide information about the effectiveness of classroom instruction.

HOW MUCH TIME DOES IT TAKE TO ADMINISTER AND SCORE WRITING CBM?

It takes approximately 5 minutes to administer a writing sample to an individual or a whole group. The time needed for scoring Writing CBM depends on the number of measures scored and the grade level of the students (the time needed increases with grade level). Malecki and Jewell (2003) found that it took an average of 30 seconds to score a single fluency measure (TWW or WSC). When two fluency measures (TWW and CWS) were scored, the time increased to a little less than a minute for elementary grades and just over a minute for middle school grades. The time increased to 1½ minutes for early elementary student levels and 2½ minutes for middle school student levels when all three measures (TWW, WSC, and CWS) were scored. If only CWS is scored, an average of 45 seconds to 1½ minutes is needed.

EXPECTED GROWTH RATES AND NORMS FOR WRITING CBM

While most content areas of CBM have established growth rates, benchmarks, or norms, there currently is no research on Writing CBM related to growth rates and benchmarks. There are norms that can be used to compare a student's score to the level of performance and rate of progress to others in his grade or instructional level. Table 6.1 provides information on norms for Writing CBM for grades 1 through 8.

HOW TO USE THE INFORMATION
TO WRITE WRITING IEP GOALS AND OBJECTIVES

Using the same format presented in Chapter 3, here are some examples of using Writing CBM data to write goals and objectives. The principles are the same: time, learner, behavior (e.g., writes), level (e.g., grade), content (e.g., writing), material (story starter CBM progress-monitoring material), and criteria (will reflect the norms or benchmarks for that skill including time and accuracy).

EXAMPLE OF GOALS

- Writing goal
  - In 30 weeks, Jose will write from sixth-grade writing story starter CBM progress-monitoring material at 47 CWS in 3 minutes with greater than 95% accuracy.

The same principles apply to writing objectives, but one should use a shorter time frame.

EXAMPLE OF OBJECTIVES

- Writing objective
  - In 10 weeks, Jose will write from sixth-grade writing story starter CBM progress-monitoring material at 30 CWS in 3 minutes with greater than 95% accuracy.

FREQUENTLY ASKED QUESTIONS ABOUT WRITING CBM

1. *What do you do if a student stops writing before the time is up?* You should say to the student: **"Keep writing the best story you can."** This prompt can be used as many times as needed.

2. *Does it matter that a student's response does not relate to the story starter?* No. Responses are not scored for content, organization, or detail. You would, however want to note this and make sure that the student understands the story starters or has the background knowledge to be able to write on the topic.

3. *Can I change the directions or how I score the student responses?* No. The directions are already short and provide you with a standard procedure to follow. Even though they may not seem to be using it productively, it is especially important to give the students 1 minute of think time before they begin to write.

TABLE 6.1. Norms for Writing CBM: Correct Writing Sequences (CWS)

Grade	Percentile	AIMSweb (2008)[a]		
		Fall (CWS)	Winter (CWS)	Spring (CWS)
1	90%	9	14	21
	75%	4	9	15
	50%	**2**	**4**	**9**
	25%	0	1	5
	10%	0	0	2
2	90%	20	30	38
	75%	13	21	29
	50%	**7**	**14**	**20**
	25%	3	8	12
	10%	1	3	6
3	90%	36	45	51
	75%	27	35	40
	50%	**17**	**24**	**29**
	25%	9	16	19
	10%	4	9	11
4	90%	48	55	64
	75%	37	45	52
	50%	**26**	**33**	**39**
	25%	16	23	28
	10%	9	15	17
5	90%	58	63	69
	75%	46	51	59
	50%	**34**	**40**	**45**
	25%	23	29	32
	10%	14	19	22
6	90%	63	70	75
	75%	52	58	63
	50%	**40**	**46**	**50**
	25%	29	34	36
	10%	19	23	25
7	90%	70	76	80
	75%	58	63	67
	50%	**44**	**50**	**52**
	25%	31	36	38
	10%	20	25	26
8	90%	77	77	82
	75%	64	66	70
	50%	**50**	**52**	**56**
	25%	36	39	42
	10%	24	26	29

[a]2008 data updated for third printing.

4. *Can I create my own story starters?* Yes, as long as they are appropriate for the grade level and elicit more than a yes/no response. This can also offer an opportunity to incorporate students' interests in the writing task.

5. *What if a student does not start writing even though I know he is capable?* Encourage the student to begin writing. Let the student know what the expectations are. If necessary, implement instructional or behavioral techniques to address the student's area of need.

6. *What if I cannot read the student's writing?* Assess if the student needs instruction in handwriting or if it is just carelessness. Then provide interventions to address the problem (e.g., handwriting practice, motivational tools, etc.). Administer additional story starters as necessary.

7. *Can students score each other's responses?* No. Students can score their own TWW, but the other measures should be scored by the teacher or someone trained in Writing CBM.

8. *Can I use student responses on Writing CBM to give grades?* This can be done if you also include an additional scoring procedure (e.g., a rubric) that looks at the content you are teaching.

9. *What should I do with the scored stories?* This information can be kept in a portfolio along with the graphed data to demonstrate progress over the year. Students can also use their responses as starting points for longer writing assignments.

10. *I only have 20 CBM story starters, but I need to progress monitor for 35 weeks. Is it OK to use the same story starters again?* Yes. Once you have used all 20, start using them again. The student probably doesn't remember specific items he did 20 weeks ago. This also means that you should not use the story starters for homework or additional practice if you want to use them again.

RESOURCES AND FURTHER READING

Espin, C. A., Scierka, B. J., Skare, S., & Halverson, N. (1999). Criterion-related validity of curriculum-based measures in writing for secondary school students. *Reading and Writing Quarterly: Overcoming Learning Difficulties, 15*(1), 5–27.

Gansle, K. A., Noell, G. H., VanDerHeyden, A. M., Naquin, G. M., & Slider, N. J. (2002). Moving beyond total words written: The reliability, criterion validity, and time cost of alternate measures for curriculum-based measurement in writing. *School Psychology Review, 31*, 477–497.

Gansle, K. A., Noell, G. H., VanDerHeyden, A. M., Slider, N. J., Hoffpauir, L. D., Whitmarsh, E. L., et al. (2004). An examination of the criterion validity and sensitivity to brief intervention of alternate curriculum-based measures of writing skill. *Psychology in the Schools, 41*, 291–300.

Lembke, E., Deno, S. L., & Hall, K. (2003). Identifying an indicator of growth in early writing proficiency for elementary school students. *Assessment for Effective Intervention, 28*(3/4), 23–35.

Malecki, C. K., & Jewell, J. (2003). Developmental, gender, and practical considerations in scoring curriculum-based measurement writing probes. *Psychology in the Schools, 40*, 379–390.

7

How to Conduct Math CBM

OVERVIEW OF WHY TO CONDUCT MATH CBM

Reading and literacy are often considered the most important skills taught in schools; however, many argue that math is similarly important for success in life. Just as for other skills, Math CBM provides a reliable and valid way to identify (1) students who are at risk for failure, (2) students who are not making adequate progress given the instruction they are receiving, (3) students who need additional diagnostic evaluation, and (4) students' instructional level. Most math assessments do not provide information about fluency, which is just as big a drawback as it is for reading since fluency provides information about skill mastery.

Math CBM is easy and efficient to administer and score. It can be administered individually or to an entire class at the same time. Math CBM can be broken down into three areas: Early Numeracy, Computation, and Concepts and Applications. Computation has been the traditional focus of Math CBM and therefore, has the most research to support its use. It was used because of the need for a quick and easy method to measure computation performance that would be reliable and relate to outcome measures. Great advances are being made with Early Numeracy, Concepts and Applications, and Estimation (an essential math skill). These will be discussed briefly later in the chapter, but the focus will be on administering, scoring, and using CBM for Computation. For the rest of the chapter, when we refer to Math CBM, we will be talking about Computation only.

Math CBM is conducted by having the student answer computational problems for 2 minutes. The teacher/examiner then counts the number of correct digits (CD). Notice that this is not correct problems, like many other math assessments use, but correct digits. We'll discuss why in the section on scoring. More importantly, the information gathered provides a database for each student so that appropriate instructional decisions can be made in a timely manner.

MATERIALS NEEDED TO CONDUCT MATH CBM

1. Different but equivalent math sheets.
2. Directions for administering and scoring Math CBM.
3. Writing utensils for student responses.
4. A stopwatch or countdown timer that displays seconds.
5. A quiet testing environment to work with students.
6. An equal-interval graph to plot the data or a graphing program

Math CBM Sheets

Other content areas such as reading or writing generally allow for generic passages, lists, or story starters. For example, reading passages at a third-grade level of difficulty are pretty similar regardless of curriculum. Math, however, often has a specific scope and sequence that can vary from state to state, school to school, and curriculum to curriculum. Many educators like to have math sheets that are linked directly to the skills included in their state's core curriculum (Why wouldn't you want to have your progress-monitoring measure aligned with the outcome measure used at the end of the year?). As such, generic or premade sheets may not include the same skills at each level. If you cannot find premade sheets that fit your curriculum (see Box 7.1 for information on where to obtain some), here is a guide for creating your own. It can also serve as a reference for judging the utility of other sheets you may consider purchasing. Creating your own sheets is more time consuming, but once it is done, you have a great and useful set of materials. To cut the workload, try to find others who can make some of the sheets for the grade level or even do some of the other grades. You can also go to one of many websites that will help you create Math CBM sheets (see Box 7.2).

The math tests used for screening, progress monitoring, and survey-level assessment usually take the form of SBMs. As you will recall from Chapter 1, SBMs consist of all the specific skills expected to be mastered by the end of the year rather than a general, cap-stone task as used in GOMs (which is what has been presented for Reading, Early Reading, and Writing CBMs in the previous chapters). The math sheets themselves should have different problems but be equivalent in difficulty (i.e., at the same grade level) and should have at least 25 problems per page (Fuchs & Fuchs, 1991) (see Figure 7.1).[1] The math problems should represent the skills the student is expected to master throughout the entire school year. This is accomplished by examining the year-long math curriculum and determining the emphasis on the skills covered during the year. Based on what skills will be taught and how much time is spent teaching each skill (an indicator of emphasis), math problems are selected or developed for each sheet. While the problems on each

---

[1]Some people use the common rule that fluency probes should contain 30–40% more items (in this case digits, not problems) than the criterion for acceptable performance (CAP). This way if a student finishes the probe, you know that she is performing well above the CAP anyway and there is not a concern about her performance. For example, mastery level (i.e., the CAP) for fourth grade is greater than 49 CD. If your fluency probes contain at least 64–69 digits, any student who finishes the probe accurately in less than 2 minutes is probably doing fine.

BOX 7.1. Where to Find Premade Math CBM Sheets

$ indicates there is a cost for the materials and/or graphing program.

⌨ indicates computerized administration available.

✍ indicates data management and graphing available.

AIMSweb (Pearson) $✍

Website: *www.aimsweb.com*

Phone: 866-323-6194

Address: Harcourt Assessment, Inc.
AIMSweb Customer Service
P.O. Box 599700
San Antonio, TX 78259

Products: • Early Numeracy (30 progress monitoring sheets, 3 benchmarking sheets for each skill)
• Computation (40 each for grades 1–8)
• Math Facts (40 each for grades 1–8)

Minneapolis Public Schools

Website: *pic.mpls.k12.mn.us/Performance_Assessment_e-Manual.html*

Products: • Computation (3 benchmarking, 7 progress monitoring sheets per grade 1–6)

MBSP Basic Math Computation—Second Edition (PRO-ED) $

Website: *www.proedinc.com/customer/ProductLists.aspx?SearchWord=MBSP*

Phone: 800-897-3202

Address: 8700 Shoal Creek Boulevard
Austin, TX 78757-6897

Products: • Computation (25 each for grades 1–6)
• Concepts and Applications (30 each for grades 2–6)

Research Institute on Progress Monitoring

Website: *progressmonitoring.org*

Phone: 612-626-7220

Products: • Early Numeracy (3 benchmarking sheets per skill)

Vanderbilt University $ (copying and postage only)

Phone: 615-343-4782

Address: Lynn Fuchs
Peabody #328
230 Appleton Place
Nashville, TN 37203-5721

(continued)

Products: • Computation (30 sheets each for grades 1–8)
         • Concepts and Applications (30 sheets each for grades 1–8)

Yearly Progress Pro (CTB/McGraw-Hill) $ 🖳 ✍

Website: *www.ctb.com/mktg/ypp/ypp_index.jsp*

Phone: 800-538-9547

Products: • Computation, Math Facts, and Concepts and Applications (sheets are
           generated from a test bank and aligned to curriculum)

BOX 7.2. Websites for Creating Math CBM Sheets

www.aplusmath.com/

Has premade single-skill sheets for computation, decimals, fractions, money, and algebra. Some also available as online sheets that are automatically scored. Also contains a worksheet generator to make mixed-math sheets.

www.interventioncentral.org/htmdocs/tools/mathprobe/addsing.shtml

Generates single-skill or mixed-math sheets. Allows detailed selection of problem types. Can be included in order selected or randomized. Also allows you to set number of rows and columns.

themathworksheetsite.com/

Can generate single-skill or mixed-math sheets. Also allows for fractions, measurement, graphing, and telling time. Not much control in creating sheets. There is also a subscription-access-only area with many other types of sheets and skills available.

superkids.com/aweb/tools/math/

Has generators for single-skill sheets and a mixed addition/subtraction version. No other mixed-math capabilities. Also has generators for fractions, greater than/less than, rounding, averages, and telling time. Provides basic, advanced (includes negative numbers and decimals), and horizontal versions for computation skills.

www.schoolhousetech.com/

Free resources include basic facts worksheet factory with addition, subtraction, multiplication, multiplication/division, and mixed options. Rather than creating sheets online, is a program to download and run on your own computer. Pay version includes many more skills and options for customizing sheets.

Math: Grade 3   Sheet 1

Name: _____   Date: _____

6	952	614	156	141
× 7	+ 768	− 44	+ 32	− 30
476	9	156	982	321
− 143	× 0	+ 284	− 97	+ 147
241	829	6	86	328
+ 118	− 106	× 0	+ 78	− 142
41	564	98	9	249
−18	+ 222	− 17	× 5	+ 92
409	728	311	256	4
+ 292	− 260	+ 188	− 45	× 1

FIGURE 7.1. Example of a mixed-math CBM sheet (student copy).

sheet should have different numerals (i.e., problems testing the same skill should contain different numbers), the number of problems representing each skill should be the same on every sheet. Therefore, each sheet is equivalent and represents the curriculum from the entire year (Fuchs & Fuchs, 1991).

For example, a third-grade curriculum might include the following math computation skills:

1. Multidigit addition without regrouping.
2. Multidigit addition with regrouping.
3. Multidigit subtraction without regrouping.
4. Multidigit subtraction with regrouping.
5. Multiplication facts, factors to 9.

If these skills appear to be equally weighted in the curriculum, we include an equal number of items for each skill on each sheet. This gives us a 5 × 5 grid to guide the construction of the 25-item sheet. Figure 7.1 is an example of what one of our third-grade math sheets might look like. Skills-based sheets such as the one in Figure 7.1 are sometimes called mixed-math sheets because they contain problems of different math computation skills that are included in the year's curriculum.

Notice that the items on the sheet are not in the order they are presented in the curriculum (i.e., multidigit addition without regrouping first, multiplication facts last). The order of the items is random so that they are not in order of increasing difficulty or complexity, but they are in a systematic order after the first line. Looking down the sheet, you can see that similar item types are grouped diagonally. This can assist us when looking for patterns in student responses to specific types of math problems. Making plans at this stage helps provide us with valuable information when using the sheets. We will discuss this in more detail later in the chapter.

Another way to create math sheets is to create sheets that test only one skill (see Figure 7.2). Single-skill math sheets should only contain problems of one operation. A single-skill sheet can be created using only the basic facts of that operation (e.g., addition facts of addends 0–9, sums 0–18 as in Figure 7.2). When a student is just beginning to learn a skill, this type of sheet can be helpful for short-term planning. A single-skill sheet can also be created using a combination of within-operation skills. For example, the sheet could contain basic facts, 2 digit × 2 digit addition without regrouping, 2 digit × 2 digit addition with regrouping, 3 digit × 3 digit addition without regrouping, 3 digit × 3 digit addition with regrouping, etc.). This type of sheet isn't appropriate for screening or progress monitoring (because it only assesses one skill), but it can be used to gain some diagnostic information or to use as a starting point for a curriculum-based evaluation (CBE) approach to decision making.

Math: Addition Facts

Name: _____   Date: _____

```
   9        1        1        3        1
 + 3      + 3      + 6      + 8      + 6

   2        1        4        6        5
 + 1      + 8      + 7      + 8      + 2

   2        8        2        3        3
 + 6      + 8      + 7      + 3      + 4

   1        5        8        8        9
 + 1      + 2      + 1      + 7      + 1

   8        1        2        6        1
 + 2      + 8      + 3      + 5      + 5
```

FIGURE 7.2. Example of a single-skill math CBM sheet (student copy).

Two copies of each math sheet will be needed: one copy for the student to write on (Figure 7.1 is an example) and one copy for the teacher/examiner that contains the correct answers and indicates the correct number of digits for each problem (see Figure 7.3). A correct digit is the right numeral in the right place (see "Directions and Scoring Procedures for Math CBM" below for specific guidelines).

The first time Math CBM materials are administered, three equivalent math sheets should be used. This can be accomplished in one testing session, but it can occur across consecutive days if needed. We recommend doing it in one session to save set-up time and obtain a more accurate score. The median score of these three samples will be used to provide the first data point on the student's graph. After that, 20–30 different but equivalent math sheets will be used to monitor student progress in math throughout the year.

Similar to the Maze CBM, Spelling CBM lists, and Writing CBM story starters, Math CBM can be administered individually or to a group. The students should have a pencil or pen and a copy of the math sheet (without the answers) in front of them, and the teacher/examiner should have a timer and the directions.

Math: Grade 3   Sheet 1

Name: _____   Date: _____

6	952	614	156	141	
× 7	+ 768	− 44	+ 32	−30	
42	**1720**	**570**	**188**	**111**	15(15)
(2)	(4)	(3)	(3)	(3)	
476	9	156	982	321	
−143	× 0	+ 284	− 97	+ 147	
333	**0**	**440**	**885**	**468**	13(28)
(3)	(1)	(3)	(3)	(3)	
241	829	6	86	328	
+ 118	− 106	× 0	+ 78	−142	
359	**723**	**0**	**164**	**186**	13(41)
(3)	(3)	(1)	(3)	(3)	
41	564	98	9	249	
− 18	+ 222	− 17	× 5	+ 92	
23	**786**	**81**	**45**	**341**	12(53)
(2)	(3)	(2)	(2)	(3)	
409	728	311	256	4	
+ 292	− 260	+ 188	− 45	× 1	
701	**468**	**499**	**211**	**4**	13(66)
(3)	(3)	(3)	(3)	(1)	

FIGURE 7.3. Example of a mixed-math CBM sheet (teacher's copy).

DIRECTIONS AND SCORING PROCEDURES FOR MATH CBM

For your convenience, Appendix B includes a reproducible version of the directions and scoring rules for Math CBM.

Directions for Math CBM[2]

1. Place a copy of the student sheet in front of the students.
2. • For single-skill sheets, say: *"The sheets on your desk have [addition, subtraction, multiplication, division, fractions, ratios, decimals, etc.] problems on them. Look at each problem carefully before you answer it. When I say, 'Please begin,' start answering the problems. Begin with the first problem and work across the page (point). Then go to the next row. If you cannot answer the problem, mark an 'X' through it and go to the next one. If you finish a page, turn the page and continue working until I say 'Thank you.' Are there any questions? Please begin."*
   • For mixed-math sheets, say: *"The sheets on your desk have math problems on them. There are several types of problems on the sheet. Some are (insert types of problems on sheet). Look at each problem carefully before you answer it. When I say 'Please begin,' start answering the problems. Begin with the first problem and work across the page (point). Then go to the next row. If you cannot answer the problem, mark an 'X' through it and go to the next one. If you finish a page, turn the page and continue working until I say 'Thank you.' Are there any questions? Please begin."*
3. Once you say **"Please begin,"** start the countdown timer (set for 2 minutes). At the end of 2 minutes, say: **"Thank you"** and have the students put their pencils down and stop working.

Scoring Math CBM

1. Count the total number of correct digits (CD).
2. Record CD for each student.

When scoring Math CBM, the number of correct digits in the solution to the problem (which includes critical processes, not just the answer) rather than the number of correct problems is used because it is a more sensitive measure to change. It is also considered a fairer metric because the student is awarded more points for correctly solving more complex problems. Since complex problems generally take more time to solve than basic ones, a greater number of points is available for the greater time commitment (this is important on a timed task).

---

[2]Adapted from Shinn (1989).

Some Math CBM programs only count the total number of correct digits in the answer. This, too, may be problematic because a division problem that has 3 CD in the answer would be worth the same number of points as an addition with 3 CD in the answer despite the additional steps (i.e., critical processes).

Figure 7.4 shows two math problems. If we were counting the number of *problems* correct, each would be worth one point. When counting the number of *digits* correct, a correct answer for the first problem (see panel A) would be worth 2 CD because that is how many are included in the longest approach to solve that problem. If a student got one of those digits wrong (e.g., wrote 40 instead of 41—see panel C), she would get credit for one digit rather than no credit for the problem. In the second example, there are 21 digits in the long version of solving the problem (see panel B). If the student did all the steps correctly except for one and got an answer of 182828 (rather than 182928), she would get credit for 20 CD (panel D). When a student makes an error in one step of a multistep solution (e.g., the second problem in Figure 7.4 has a transcription error in the answer—the student wrote 8 instead of 9 even though she did all the work correctly), if the scoring is by digit, she is only penalized for the one digit that is incorrect. If the scoring were by problem, she would get no credit. For each math problem, the number of correct digits is counted and then added together to get the total number of CD. For the student to get credit for a CD it must be the right digit in the right place.

Scored as Correct

- If the student has the correct answer, she is given credit for the longest method used to solve the problem *even if all the work is not shown*. If the student gets the

A	B
$\begin{array}{r} 25 \\ + 16 \\ \hline 41 \end{array}$ 2 CD	$\begin{array}{r} 1236 \\ \times 148 \\ \hline 9888 \\ 49440 \\ 123600 \\ \hline 182928 \end{array}$ 21 CD
C	D
$\begin{array}{r} 25 \\ + 16 \\ \hline 4\cancel{0} \end{array}$ 1 CD	$\begin{array}{r} 1236 \\ \times 148 \\ \hline 9888 \\ 49440 \\ 123600 \\ \hline 182\cancel{8}28 \end{array}$ 20 CD

FIGURE 7.4. Sample math problems with correct digits.

correct answer, she has demonstrated that she knows how to solve the problem and, therefore, gets full credit.

```
        1236              1236
      × 148              × 148
       9888            182928
      49440
     123600
     182928

      21 CD              21 CD
```

- If a problem has been crossed out or started, but not completed, the student still receives credit for any correct digits. Correct work is correct work, even if the student did not finish the problem.

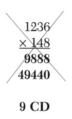

9 CD

- Reversed or rotated digits are scored as correct with the exception of 6's and 9's. With 6's and 9's, it is not possible to tell which one the student meant to write. No other digits can become others through rotation or reversal.

```
        25                 25
      + 16               + 16
        41                ↩ 1

      2 CD               2 CD
```

- In multiplication problems, any symbol used as a place holder is counted as a correct digit as long as it is holding a place that needs to be held. The student can use a 0, X, ☺, a blank space, or whatever else as long as it is used to hold that place.

```
        1236              1236
      × 148              × 148
       9888              9888
      49440             4944x
     123600            123600
     182928            182928

      21 CD             21 CD
```

Scored as Errors

All errors are marked with a slash (/). See Figure 7.4 for two examples.

Special Scoring Examples

- Parts of the answer above the line, such as carries or borrows, are not counted as correct digits. These are part of the work of the solution—not the solution itself—thus, their correctness is shown in the answer below the line.

	124
1236	1236
× 148	× 148
9888	9888
49440	49440
123600	123600
182928	182928
21 CD	**21 CD**

- In division, a basic fact is when both the divisor and the quotient are 9 or less. The total CD is always 1. Also, remainders of 0 are not counted as correct digits nor are placeholders.

$$8\overline{)24}^{\ 3} \qquad 3\overline{)9}^{\ 3}$$

Special Administration and Scoring Considerations for MATH CBM

If the student finishes in less than 2 minutes, note the number of seconds it took to complete the math sheet, and prorate the score. The formula for prorating is:

$$\frac{\text{Total number of correct digits}}{\text{Number of seconds it took to finish}} \times 120 = \text{Estimated number of correct digits in 2 minutes}$$

Example: The student finished the math sheet in just 110 seconds and got 40 digits correct.

$$\frac{40}{110} \times 120 = 0.36 \times 120 = 43.6$$

We estimate that the student would have completed approximately 44 correct digits in 2 minutes had we provided more problems and timed her for the full 2 minutes.

HOW OFTEN SHOULD MATH CBM BE GIVEN?

In Chapter 3, we provide additional details on how often and when to administer CBM for the different purposes of screening/benchmarking, progress monitoring, and survey-level assessment. Below we provide only an outline for these purposes. We suggest you refer to Chapter 3 for a more in-depth discussion on how often and when to give CBM for these different purposes.

- Screening/benchmarking = all students in a classroom or grade level, once per quarter (three to four times per school year); typically conducted in the fall, winter, and spring.
- Progress monitoring = students in the bottom 25% of the class based on the screening assessment, at least one time per week—preferably two times per week. This includes any student who is considered at risk based on norms or benchmark criteria.
- Monthly progress monitoring of all students can provide information about the effectiveness of classroom instruction.
- Survey-level assessment = students who will be progress monitored; this could be done at the beginning of the year, during benchmarking, or anytime throughout the school year. Conducting SLA can be streamlined if it is done along with benchmarking since you will already have three examples of student work. This is also helpful when a teacher has a student enter his classroom in between benchmarking periods.

HOW MUCH TIME DOES IT TAKE TO ADMINISTER AND SCORE MATH CBM?

The time needed to score each student sheet is the same for single-skill or mixed-math Math CBM. If you are giving a test to a class of 25 students or an individual student the time is still 2 minutes for the test itself plus the time to get the students ready and for them to hand in their work. We would estimate this process, once the students are familiar with it, should take from 5 to 10 minutes to administer the test.

Knowing the number of CD for each problem and row and for the total sheet will assist in scoring. It will not be necessary to count the CD for each problem if they are all calculated correctly. If the student misses only a few CD, you can subtract the difference from the total CD as opposed to adding the CD for each problem. As with most things, you will become more proficient with practice. We estimate that it would take no longer than 1–2 minutes to score CD for each student.

EXPECTED GROWTH RATES AND NORMS FOR MATH CBM

How Much Progress Can We Expect in Math?

Once the CD for each problem has been added up, the next step is to determine how much progress should be made on a weekly basis. Table 7.1 provides information on expected growth for Math CBM for grades 1 through 6. Once the amount of progress is determined, the goal can also be determined and drawn on the student's graph. The usual cautions about setting progress goals in this fashion apply. Remember that rates of progress are not ceilings and that greater progress may be possible. Also, if a student is not making adequate progress, this does not mean that she lacks the ability to learn math. It means the instruction may need to be changed. A diagnostic evaluation may also be needed. This is all discussed in more detail in Chapter 8.

Proficiency Levels or Benchmarks for Math CBM

In addition to having a standard to compare a student's weekly growth to (i.e., her rate of progress), it is important to have standards for level of performance. These are often referred to as benchmarks. While a lot of work has been done to determine benchmarks for Reading and Early Reading CBM tasks, much less has been done with Math. The top section of Table 7.2 shows the original placement levels proposed by Deno and Mirkin (1977). These levels have never been empirically validated. Burns, VanDerHeyden, and Jiban (2006) have recently done work to validate those levels. Their preliminary data are shown in the bottom part of Table 7.2.

Norms for Math CBM

Another way to set standards for performance is to compare a student's score to the performance of others in her grade or instructional level. These norms have been collected over numerous years and from numerous sources. It should be mentioned that they have not been collected in a traditional sense, making sure that the students in the norm group

TABLE 7.1. Weekly Growth Rates for Math CBM: Correct Digits (CD)

Grade	Realistic growth rates per week (CD)	Ambitious growth rates per week (CD)
1	0.30	0.50
2	0.30	0.50
3	0.30	0.50
4	0.70	1.15
5	0.75	1.20
6	0.45	1.00

Note. Data from Fuchs, Fuchs, Hamlett, Walz, and Germann (1993).

TABLE 7.2. Benchmarks for Math CBM: Correct Digits (CD)

Grade level	Placement level	CD
Data from Deno and Mirkin (1977).		
1–3	Frustration	< 20
	Instructional	21–40
	Mastery	> 41
4–12	Frustration	< 40
	Instructional	41–80
	Mastery	> 81
Data from Burns, VanDerHeyden, and Jiban (2006).		
2–3	Frustration	< 14
	Instructional	14–31
	Mastery	> 31
4–5	Frustration	< 24
	Instructional	24–49
	Mastery	> 49

have similar characteristics to the U.S. population as determined using the U.S. Census. It is interesting to note, however, that the data have been collected on thousands of students across the country and the numbers are very similar. This adds credibility that these norms provide a good indication of how students perform (see Table 7.3).

SURVEY-LEVEL ASSESSMENT WITH MATH CBM

You may remember survey-level assessment (SLA) from Chapter 3 (if not, you may want to go refresh your memory). Math CBM is the other content area where SLA has been used. The procedures are similar except that while SLA for reading uses GOMs (ORF CBM is the task used), Math CBM uses SBMs. So rather than testing forward or backward through a curriculum to find an instructional level (which still could be done using Math CBM—for example, if a student was new to a classroom and the teacher had no records on her previous performance), SLA for math is done slightly differently.

The first step is to administer three sheets at the appropriate curriculum level (generally the student's grade level). Record the scores and grade level in the "Mixed Math" table in the SLA Math sheet. A reproducible version of this form is available in Appendix B. Find the median CD and compare that score to the performance criteria. If the student's performance is in the instructional range, great; if it is in the frustrational range, the teacher should administer single-skill sheets that correspond to the skills included in the mixed-math sheets just administered. If sheets have been set up to provide preliminary diagnostic information, the teacher will have an idea of which skills to focus on.

TABLE 7.3. Norms for Math CBM:
Correct Digits (CD)

Grade	Percentile	AIMSweb (2008)[a] Fall (CD)	Winter (CD)	Spring (CD)
1	90%	11	22	28
	75%	8	16	20
	50%	**5**	**11**	**15**
	25%	2	7	10
	10%	0	4	6
2	90%	19	35	41
	75%	14	29	31
	50%	**10**	**22**	**22**
	25%	7	15	16
	10%	5	10	11
3	90%	27	39	46
	75%	21	31	37
	50%	**15**	**24**	**28**
	25%	11	18	21
	10%	9	12	15
4	90%	60	76	87
	75%	45	60	70
	50%	**33**	**44**	**52**
	25%	24	33	38
	10%	16	23	27
5	90%	48	60	71
	75%	39	49	60
	50%	**30**	**38**	**47**
	25%	23	28	35
	10%	16	19	25
6	90%	51	65	66
	75%	38	49	50
	50%	**28**	**36**	**34**
	25%	21	26	26
	10%	16	20	20

[a]2008 data updated for third printing.

HOW TO USE THE INFORMATION
TO WRITE MATH IEP GOALS AND OBJECTIVES

Using the same format presented in Chapter 3, here are some examples of using Math CBM data to write goals and objectives. The principles are the same: time, learner, behavior (e.g., calculates, adds, subtracts), level (e.g., grade), content (e.g., math), material (Math CBM progress-monitoring material), and criteria (will reflect the norms or benchmarks for that skill including time and accuracy).

EXAMPLE OF GOALS

- Math goal
  - In 30 weeks, Larry will calculate addition and subtraction problems from second-grade mixed-math CBM progress-monitoring material at 45 CD in 2 minutes with greater than 95% accuracy.

The same principles apply to writing objectives, but one should use a shorter time frame.

EXAMPLE OF OBJECTIVES

- Math objective
  - In 10 weeks, Larry will calculate addition and subtraction problems from second-grade mixed-math CBM progress-monitoring material at 20 CD in 2 minutes with greater than 95% accuracy.

SPECIAL CONSIDERATIONS THAT APPLY TO MATH CBM

Accuracy of Teacher/Examiner Copy

Because the teacher's/examiner's copy is invaluable and time saving, it is critically important that it is correct. This sounds like common sense, but it is very important to make sure that the answers to the problems and the number of correct digits assigned to them are all correct—*even if you have gotten premade sheets.* One of us was using a set of premade sheets downloaded for free. One of the forms had been used about five or six times before a scoring error was noticed. The error reduced the CD for one problem by 2. This may not seem like much, but when comparing that sheet to others (such as during progress monitoring), it will systematically underestimate a student's performance.

Setting Up Math CBM Sheets to Provide Potential Diagnostic Information

Unlike reading or writing, math is easier to separate into discrete skills. Therefore, when developing math sheets, it is prudent to plan so that the results can be used in a diagnostic way. Take our example of aligning the math sheet with our curriculum. We were able to identify five skills that needed to be included. Our sheet was easily set up into five columns and five rows, giving us a total of 25 problems. We then took each of those five skills and put them on a diagonal (see Figure 7.5). This way, as we score the sheet, we can look to see if there is a pattern of the student missing problems within a diagonal. If the student misses all of the problems in a diagonal, we should check to see if the student has been taught that skill yet. If so, it might be one that the student needs additional instruction on or practice with. We could also look to determine if the student has difficulty with the basic facts that support a certain skill or multiple skills. This is often the case when

Math: Grade 3   Sheet 1

Name: _____   Date: _____

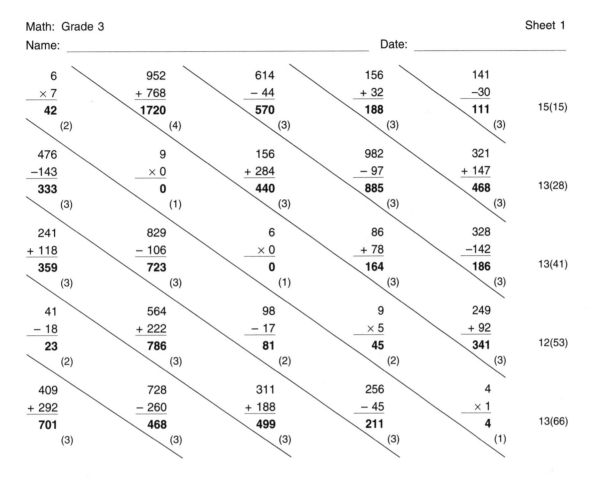

FIGURE 7.5. Example of a mixed-math CBM sheet set up for diagnostic decision making.

the student has difficulty doing multidigit problems that involve borrowing or carrying (although it might also be an issue of place value or the process of borrowing/carrying). Again, these patterns should not be considered reliable evidence of that student's deficit in the specific skills, but should be considered as hypotheses to test with more in-depth measures (such as a single-skill sheet) or evidence of skills that need to be taught or reviewed. (The adage we like to adhere to is "When in doubt, teach.")

Early Numeracy

Just as early literacy skills have gained in prominence for assessment of reading (in order to prevent future problems), early numeracy skills are gaining prominence in math. Research on Early Numeracy CBM is in its infancy, but there are several promising measures. A brief overview is provided here, but for further information turn to the "Resources and Further Reading" section. Figure 7.6 includes examples of Early Numeracy CBM tasks.

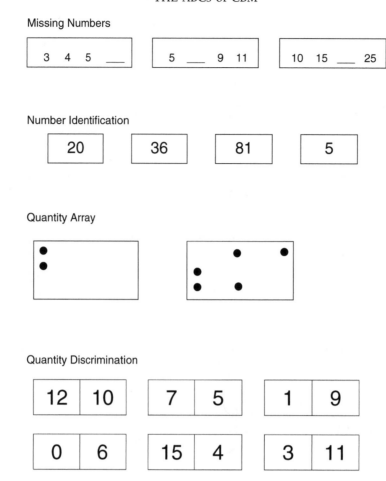

FIGURE 7.6. Early numeracy skills and sample problems.

Missing Numbers

For this measure, the student is presented with a box that contains three numbers and a blank. The numbers have a pattern to them (either counting by 1's, 2's, 5's, or 10's). The student is to tell the teacher/examiner the number that correctly completes the pattern (i.e., fits in the blank). This measure must be administered individually and takes 1 minute.

Number Identification

For this measure, the student is presented with a sheet of numbers (0–100 or 0–20, depending on the source of the sheets) in random order. The student tells the teacher/ examiner what each number is. The measure must be administered individually and takes 1 minute.

Oral Counting

For this measure, the student counts orally starting at one. The teacher/examiner scores on a sheet of the numbers from 1 to 100. The measure must be administered individually and takes 1 minute.

Quantity Array

For this measure, the student is presented with a box containing several dots. The student is to identify how many dots are in each box and tell the teacher/examiner. The measure must be administered individually and takes 1 minute.

Quantity Discrimination

For this measure, the student is presented with two adjoining boxes that each contain a number. The student is to identify which number is greater and tell the teacher/examiner. The measure must be administered individually and takes 1 minute.

Concepts and Applications

A problem many people have with using computation as the sole skill measured by Math CBM is that, especially in the older grades, there is a lot more to math than computation. Therefore, Math CBM has been extended to include other math skills. The Concepts and Applications sheets used by the National Center on Progress Monitoring include other math skills, such as measurement, time, graph interpretation, and many others found in math curriculums. These measures deviate from traditional CBM in a few ways. First, the response format varies—some items are fill in the blank; others are multiple choice. Second, the first-grade measure is read to the student, but all others are completed independently. Because there is reading involved in this math assessment, reading the measure to the students attempts to reduce the effect of reading on the student's performance. Third, the time to complete each sheet is 6–8 minutes as compared to the 2 minutes for Computation or 1 minute for Early Numeracy. Because the skills are more complex and varied, extra time is needed; however, this does make use of the measure more time consuming.

Estimation

One of the concepts included in the Concepts and Applications measure is estimation. This is an important math skill that is being explored as a useful criterion measure because it is thought to be a good indicator of number sense. Estimation sheets generally consist of 40 problems (both word and computation format) with three answers provided. One of the answers is close to the correct answer (how close it is varies) but not exact, and the other two are further away. Students are to identify which of the provided answers is closest to the correct answer. They have 3 minutes to complete as many of the problems as possible.

FREQUENTLY ASKED QUESTIONS ABOUT MATH CBM

1. *Do teachers generally administer Math CBM sheets one-on-one with each student or to a group?* It depends on the teacher and the purpose. When screening a whole class, it makes more sense to administer to the entire group. When doing weekly progress monitoring, you might do it individually or with a small group of two to three students.

2. *My student has improved her math performance as I have monitored her progress, but she is not receiving any instruction in math. Could assessing using CBM alone be making a difference?* The extra 2 minutes of practice that she is getting per week is probably not enough to show improvement. She may be practicing elsewhere or receiving additional instruction.

3. *I only have 20 Math CBM sheets, but I need to progress monitor for 35 weeks. Is it OK to use the same sheets again?* Yes. Once you have used all 20, start using them again. The student probably doesn't remember specific items she did 20 weeks ago. This also means that you should not use the math sheets as homework or additional practice if you want to use them again.

4. *Should I tell my students that they get credit for each part of the computation problems rather than just correct/incorrect for the problem?* No, because it's the answer that is the most important part. If a student is concentrating on the intermediate stages even though she can calculate a complex problem in her head, she may show work she doesn't need to. This would slow her down by adding unnecessary steps. You want to get the most authentic measure of the student's performance.

5. *Because Math CBM measures fluency, skipping time-consuming problems might be a calculated choice so that the student can move on to problems that can be solved more quickly. Does not answering specific questions really indicate a gap in skills or could it be a logical strategy?* More complex problems have more CD associated with them, so it's a flawed strategy anyway. If a student is skipping certain types of problems, you should administer a single-skill sheet to determine if she can't or won't do that type of problem. Sometimes the solution is as simple as asking the student, "Why did you skip these problems?" If her answer is "So I could finish more of the easier ones," you should remind her to attempt every problem and have her do another sheet.

6. *Can I use benchmark scores on Math CBM to put students in instructional groups?* Yes, if you have students with similar instructional needs. These groups should be flexible and students should be evaluated and regrouped every 6–8 weeks.

7. *Not everyone in my class is on the same instructional level. Should I still give them all the same Math CBM sheets?* All students should be screened/benchmarked on their grade level, but they should be progress monitored on their instructional level, especially if they are receiving instruction on that level. The best way to handle this is to give both the grade-level and the instructional-level math sheets each week so that you have an indication of how students are doing given the instruction they are receiving (instructional level) and how well it is transferring to more difficult problems (grade level).

8. *What should I do with the scored sheets?* This information can be kept in a portfolio along with the graphed data to demonstrate progress over the year.

RESOURCES AND FURTHER READING

Clarke, B., & Shinn, M. (2004). A preliminary investigation into the identification and development of early mathematics curriculum-based measurement. *School Psychology Review, 33,* 234–248.

Foegen, A. (2000). Technical adequacy for general outcome measures for middle school mathematics. *Diagnostique, 25,* 175–203.

Foegen, A., & Deno, S. L. (2001). Identifying growth indicators for low-achieving students in middle school mathematics. *The Journal of Special Education, 35,* 4–16.

Fuchs, L. S., Fuchs, D., Hamlett, C. L., Phillips, N. B., & Bentz, J. (1994). Classwide curriculum-based measurement: Helping general educators meet the challenge of student diversity. *Exceptional Children, 60,* 518–537.

Fuchs, L. S., Fuchs, D., Hamlett, C. L., & Stecker, P. M. (1990). The role of skills analysis in curriculum-based measurement in math. *School Psychology Review, 19,* 6–22.

Fuchs, L. S., Fuchs, D., Hamlett, C. L., Thompson, A., Roberts, P. H., Kubek, P., et al. (1994). Technical features of a mathematics concepts and applications curriculum-based measurement system. *Diagnostique, 19*(4), 23–49.

Thurber, R. S., Shinn, M. R., & Smolkowski, K. (2002). What is measured in mathematics tests? Construct validity of curriculum-based mathematics measures. *School Psychology Review, 31,* 498–513.

VanDerHeyden, A. M., & Burns, M. K. (2005). Using curriculum-based assessment and curriculum-based measurement to guide elementary mathematics instruction: Effect on individual and group accountability scores. *Assessment for Effective Intervention, 30,* 15–31.

8

Charting and Graphing Data
to Help Make Decisions

Getting assessment data into a form that is easy to interpret and use is one of the most important things to consider. If the data we collect are not easy to use, we will be less likely to use them, and if we do not use them, why bother collecting them? One of the main benefits of CBM is that the data are displayed in graphs and charts (which are a lot easier to read and interpret than a page full of numbers). Different types of graphs can be used to examine the data in different ways. This chapter demonstrates some types of graphs that are commonly used to display CBM data and some decision rules for using them.

PROCEDURES AND MATERIALS NEEDED TO CHART CBM DATA

The standard graph used with CBM is a typical line graph like the one in Figure 8.1. The vertical axis of the graph (marked as "Words Read Correctly"—the abscissa, for you math-o-philes) indicates the number correct on a CBM probe. The actual metric will be different for different content areas (e.g., WRC is the ORF metric for Reading CBM). The increments should be sized so that student growth can be accurately observed. Increments that are too large may understate the student's growth, and increments that are too small may overstate it. The horizontal axis (marked as "# of weeks"—the ordinate) is used to indicate the number of weeks the student will be monitored, allowing for data to be entered one to two times per week.

Because the chart has both a time axis (number of weeks) and a skill axis (WRC), it allows us to record changes in student learning over time. Learning (or a lack of it) is what we begin to see as we collect a series of data points. This is significant because it means that by charting CBM results we get two kinds of data: data on student level of

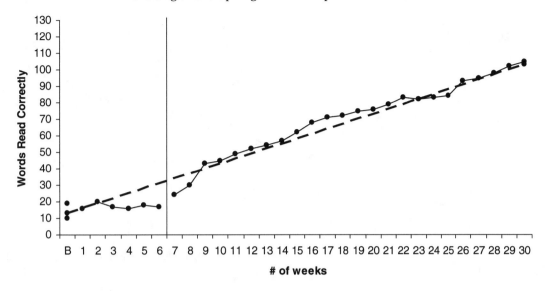

FIGURE 8.1. A typical CBM line graph.

performance, and data on student rate of progress. Performance scores tell us how well a student can do that task. Progress scores tell us how quickly she is learning how to perform it.

For each content area, the same graph should be used for each student. Figure 8.2 illustrates why. The two graphs in Figure 8.2 use the same student data. Because the vertical axis of the graph on the right only goes from 0 to 30, the student appears to be making good progress (i.e., the trend of his progress is quite steep). When we examine his progress on the graph with the vertical axis that goes from 0 to 130, it doesn't look so good. In actuality, his progress is below his peers', and the decision should be that he is *not* making adequate progress.

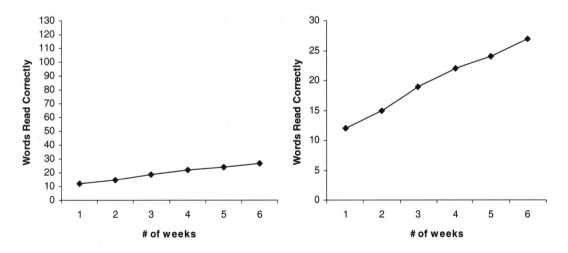

FIGURE 8.2. Student data plotted on graphs with different vertical axes.

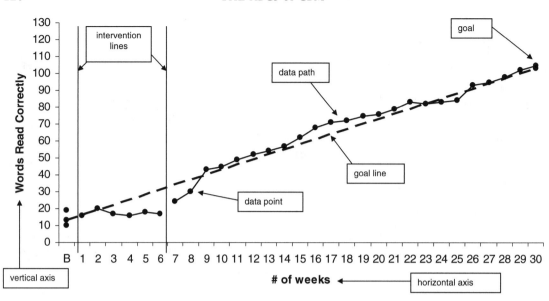

FIGURE 8.3. Sample CBM graph with each part labeled.

Figure 8.3 is an example of a CBM graph with each part of the graph labeled. The first thing we enter on the graph is the student's baseline data (the first column on the left side of the graph—marked with a B). This lets us know where the student is starting with his performance. To find the student's baseline, we administer three separate passages, lists, story starters, or sheets. Plot all three on the first vertical line. The one in the middle is the baseline score (if two scores are the same, that score is the baseline). Figure 8.3 shows that the three scores the student earned are 10, 13, and 19. His baseline score is therefore 13—the point we will start from.

HOW TO SET AND GRAPH GOALS

Now that we have plotted the student's baseline data, we need to set a goal. There are three methods to setting goals: end-of-year benchmarks, norms (national or local), and intraindividual framework. Which method to use depends on the availability of information (Are there national norms?), the student's performance level (typically performing or at risk), and the comparison you want to make (to a performance criterion or a representative peer group).

End-of-Year Benchmarks

The use of performance standards (i.e., benchmarks) is one method of determining goals. Table 3.4 in Chapter 3 shows benchmarks for grades 1 through 6 for ORF CBM. At the end of the year, we want every student to be performing at or above the benchmark. For example, for a student in third grade, we would set our end-of-year goal at 110 WRC. This is the lowest score we would accept that would indicate a student is *not* at risk for future academic failure. Even if the students were not performing at an acceptable level at the beginning of the year (when we screened/benchmarked the class), as long as they make progress that will take them to mastery by the end of the year, we can feel confident that they will be performing proficiently and will not be at risk for difficulty in reading.

Norms

Another way to set goals is to use some type of normative comparison group. There has been some work identifying national norms for CBM in most content areas. When they are available, national norms are good to use. If they are not, it is possible to develop local norms by administering the measures to every student in a school or district (or a random sample of 100 per grade level) three times per year. These scores are used to calculate local norms and should be updated every 3–5 years. This is a time-consuming practice, so we recommend using national norms whenever possible.

As mentioned in Chapter 2, it may make sense to randomly sample a small group of students and compare their scores to the norms that have already been validated. If they are similar, there is nothing to gain by generating local norms. Also, if school norms are lower than national ones, teachers would not want to use the local ones because they might give a false impression of student proficiency.

Norms come in two forms: levels of performance and rates of progress. Because CBM has been used for more than 25 years, there have been some efforts to collect large samples of scores that are representative of the U.S. school population. Others have collected large sets of data based on who is using their CBM product. These may not be truly representative, but the results seem to be quite similar. To set goals using this type of norm, you use the same process as with end-of-year benchmarks. The difference is that these are based on typical performance of same-grade peers rather than a criterion for proficiency that predicts performance on outcome measures (which is what benchmarks do). One finds the grade level the student is in, identifies the level of performance for the 50th percentile in the spring, and uses that as the end-of-year goal. The content chapters contain tables of these national sets of norms for Reading CBM (Tables 3.5 and 3.6), Early Reading CBM (Table 4.3), Spelling CBM (Table 5.2), Writing CBM (Table 6.1), and Math CBM (Table 7.3).

The other type of norm is rate of growth or progress. In addition to identifying the level of performance for national groups, some researchers have identified the typical rate of growth for large samples of students. This has been calculated as an average weekly gain. Using this weekly growth rate, you can simply multiply the rate by the number of weeks left until the aim date (i.e., the date by which you expect the student to reach the goal) for your student and add that number to his baseline score. Tables 3.2, 3.3, 5.1, and 7.1 contain the rate of growth norms for Reading (both ORF and Maze), Spelling, and Math CBM respectively. For example, assume we are working with a student in second grade whose baseline ORF score is 28 WRC. We have 20 weeks left in the school year. Setting an "ambitious" goal (see Box 8.1) using an increase of 2 WRC per week would indicate a goal of $20 \times 2 = 40 + 28 = 68$. Our goal is 68 WRC at the end of 20 weeks. This would be enough to have the student performing in the mastery range—exactly where we want him to be.

We need to note a few things about progress norms. First, progress norms reflect the quality of instruction—more intense instruction should lead to greater growth. One thing we don't know about national progress norms is how good or intense the instruction was that the students were receiving. Second, the students who are farthest behind need to have the steepest slopes (i.e., the greatest rates of progress) in order to catch up to the expected level of performance. This means they need the most intense and effective interventions.

Intraindividual Framework

Setting goals using the intraindividual framework uses the student's current level of performance and rate of progress to set end-of-the-year goals for his performance. After collecting at least eight data points, subtract the lowest score from the highest. For example, if we were progress monitoring a second-grade student using ORF passages, his first eight scores might be 12, 16, 15, 19, 16, 21, 26, and 24. We find the difference: $26 - 12 = 14$. Divide this difference by the number of weeks (i.e., the number of data points we have collected, eight): $14 \div 8 = 1.75$. This baseline rate of growth is multiplied by 1.5 in order to set a weekly progress goal: $1.75 \times 1.5 = 2.625$. This number is then multiplied by the number of weeks left until the end of the year (or the end of the planned intervention: 2.625×16 weeks $= 42$. This number is then added to the median score of the first eight data points we used to calculate the baseline growth rate (it is 17.5—halfway between 16 and 19): $42 + 17.5 = 59.5$. This is our end-of-year performance goal for this student: 59.5 (using 60 WRC as the goal ensures he scored above the goal).

While this method can be used, we caution that it may underestimate a student's rate of learning and may never catch him up if he started out behind. (Because he wasn't performing as well as he needed to is why we were concerned in the first place, right?) If the

---

BOX 8.1. Should I Use Ambitious or Realistic Goals?

The terms *ambitious* and *realistic* can be a little misleading. The term *realistic* is used to label the typical growth rate for the sample used. *Ambitious* is used to label the typical growth rate for the sample used plus 1 standard deviation (i.e., if you expressed each student's slope as a single number, typical growth is at the 50th percentile and ambitious growth is at the 84th). These values are not meant to be maximum possibilities. It isn't unrealistic to expect greater rates of growth from a student—especially if he is starting well below the typical performance. In that case, the student *must* make extraordinary growth in order to catch up to his peers. That's ambitious, but sometimes it is realistic to be ambitious.

instruction is good and the student responds positively to it, using benchmarks or norms may provide better goals since they represent scores that are predictive of future academic success (i.e., benchmarks) or an indication of how other students in that grade level perform (i.e., norms). In our opinion, the only time you would want to use a student's past performance as a goal for future performance is when his past performance is average or above average.

Graphing Goals

Now that we have set the goal for our student, we need to graph that goal on his chart. Whichever method we used to set the goal, we should have a specific target to work toward and a number of weeks we expect it will take to get there. These are the only two numbers we need to graph the student's goal. We also need to make sure that the paper we are using has enough room horizontally for all the weeks of data we will be collecting and enough room vertically to record the student's performance all the way to the goal.

Look at Figure 8.3 again. We had already plotted our student's baseline data and found his baseline score to be 13. Say we have decided to use the norm approach and set an ambitious growth rate of 3 WRC per week. Since we are planning to monitor the progress of the student's performance for the entire school year, we have 30 weeks left. So 30 weeks times 3 WRC per week is 90 WRC. In 30 weeks, we expect the student to *increase* his WRC by 90. This means we add it to his baseline score (13). At week 30 on our chart, we draw an X or a target at 103 (90 + 13). We then connect the baseline score and the goal. This is the student's goal line (also sometimes referred to as an *aimline*).

Each week, as we administer at least one passage or probe to the student, we enter his score on the graph and connect it to the previous point. These are data points and the data path. This allows each student to have his database, which is used to evaluate the effectiveness of the instruction he is receiving.

HOW OFTEN SHOULD DATA BE COLLECTED?

How frequently to collect data and graph them depends on three things. First, it depends on our purpose—is it to screen/benchmark or progress monitor? If we are assessing and graphing to screen/benchmark all students' progress, we typically use CBM measures three or four times per year. This is the "checking vital signs" exercise designed to pick up potential problems but not to yield much information about how to correct those problems when they are found. This sort of testing doesn't need to be done often. If we are monitoring progress to guide instruction, we need frequent feedback, so more frequent measurement is needed.

Second, how frequently we collect and graph data depends on the importance of the task. High-importance tasks need frequent monitoring. If there are particular skills that are of great importance, we should monitor them more directly and frequently than we would monitor skills of lesser consequence (this is basically why we watch young children more closely when they are playing near a street than when they are playing in a fenced backyard). Reading and language are good examples of skill areas in which we can't afford to let students fall behind without noticing. Reading Roman numerals might not meet the same criterion.

Third, frequency of collecting and graphing data depends on the significance of a problem. As the student's difficulties increase and the need for effective instruction becomes more urgent, the need for more frequent monitoring is increased. The magnitude of a student's difficulty is illustrated by the size of the difference between his actual level of performance and the expected level of performance as well as his rate of progress. A student who is far behind but making rapid progress may actually be seen as having less of a problem than another student who is only moderately behind expectations but making little or no progress.

What this means is that while there are no hard and fast rules for the frequency of progress monitoring, it should be increased when the content is important and the student is at risk for future academic problems. Most people recommend screening/benchmarking three or four times per year on CBM measures. Progress monitoring should be done one to two times per week for the students having the greatest difficulty and every other week to once per month for students who are not having as much difficulty. For students who are performing and progressing well, the screening/benchmarking measures may be enough to monitor their progress.

DECISION RULES TO HELP EDUCATORS USE THE DATA TO INFORM INSTRUCTION

Notice that in Figure 8.3 there are also vertical lines that seem to separate sections of the data. These are called *intervention lines*. Where an intervention line falls, the data points on either side are not connected by a data path. This is to help us remember that something changed at that point and to group the data points more easily. Each intervention line shows us the point at which a decision about the student's progress was made.

There are two methods of making decisions about whether the student's response to instruction is appropriate or not (i.e., if the student's progress is adequate for him to meet his goal within the expected time period). The first is data point analysis and the second is trend line analysis. With either method, the goal line is used as a reference point.

To use data point analysis, the data points on the graph for each week are examined. After collecting an initial six to eight data points, any time four *consecutive* scores fall below the goal line, a decision needs to be made. This decision is usually some sort of change in instruction—even something as simple as "Maybe I could meet with him earlier in the day." Lowering the goal is not considered an appropriate option. Whenever the student achieves four *consecutive* data points above the goal line, the goal is raised (see Fuchs et al., 1989). Using the data in this way allows the teacher to determine if the student is making appropriate progress or if a change in instruction is warranted. If data are not collected frequently, several weeks could go by before these rules could be applied.

The second method, trend line analysis, represents the student's *observed* rate of progress, which can be compared to the *expected* rate of progress as indicated by the goal line. The five steps below describe the Tukey method of trend line analysis.

1. Collect at least seven or eight CBM scores.
2. Divide them as evenly as possible into three groups. For example, if we collected eight data points, we might divide them into the first three, the next two, and the last three.
3. Find the median (middle) score for the first group and the last group and mark them with an X.
4. Draw a line between the two X's.
5. Compare this trend line to the goal line.

Figure 8.4 shows what this process might look like. After 8 weeks of monitoring our student's progress once per week, we have enough data points to draw a trend line. First, we group the first three data points together, the next two, and the last three. Next, we draw an X at the median point of both the first and last three data points. Notice that the X is at the midpoint both vertically (the middle score) and horizontally (the middle time point). The X shouldn't be drawn exactly *on* the middle score unless it occurred at the middle time point for that group. Last, connect the two X's and compare the trend line to the goal line.

If the trend line and goal line are similar, the student is making adequate progress. If the trend line indicates that the student will not be able to reach his goal in the time frame graphed, then instructional changes should be considered. This should be done every seven to eight data points to ensure the student is staying on track. If the trend line is consistently above the goal line, we should consider increasing the goal.

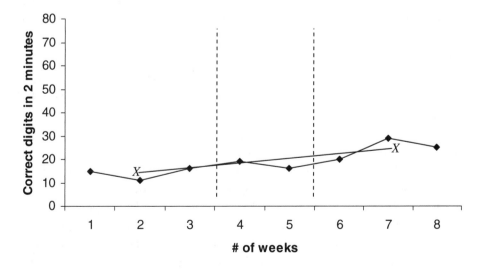

FIGURE 8.4. Example of the Tukey method of drawing a trend line.

CONSIDERATIONS FOR GRAPHING AND CHARTING
THE DATA IN THE CONTENT AREAS

The procedures for graphing are the same no matter what content area you are monitoring the student's progress in. The different expected levels of performance and rates of growth for different content areas as well as different grades can be seen in the following tables:

- Chapter 3: Reading—Tables 3.2–3.6
- Chapter 4: Early Reading—Tables 4.2 and 4.3
- Chapter 5: Spelling—Tables 5.1 and 5.2
- Chapter 6: Writing—Table 6.1
- Chapter 7: Math—Tables 7.1–7.3

It is possible to use different scales on graphs for different content areas; however, if you are trying to make comparisons across areas, this may make it confusing. For example, the graphs in Figure 8.2 could be for different content areas. Using these two graphs, you could easily make different conclusions about the student's progress in the different areas, but if you have the student's goal line plotted on each (and you should), you will have a reference point. As such, it may not be a big deal to use different vertical axes for different content areas. We recommend using the same vertical axis for all students in the same content area so that you can make accurate comparisons among students (if you are so inclined) or among grades for the same student.

THE USE OF CBM IN RESPONSE TO INTERVENTION

You've probably heard of the term *response to intervention*, or RTI; at the very least, you should have read our brief reference to it in Chapter 1. There are different approaches to RTI, but all include the use of data to make decisions about the effectiveness of instruction with students.

RTI uses a tiered approach to instruction. Tier I is the general instruction provided to all students. Tier II adds supplemental instruction for those students who are not making adequate progress with only the Tier I instruction. Tier III encompasses the most intensive instruction for those students having the greatest difficulties. The same CBM measures are used with all students across the various tiers of instruction; the only thing that really changes is the frequency of assessment. The students who need the most intensive interventions (Tier III), also need to have their progress monitored most frequently (in addition to screening/benchmarking)—one to two times per week. Students receiving supplemental instruction (i.e., Tier II) would need to have their progress monitored less frequently—every other week or once per month. The students making adequate progress with the general instruction (Tier I) are monitored even less frequently—once per month or only using the screening/benchmarking assessments of three to four times per year. These data are used to make instructional decisions.

When making decisions, one of the most important parts is to determine an appropriate standard to compare student performance to. Once you have identified the appropriate comparison, you have a basis for making judgments. We have already explained how standards for level of performance and rate of progress can be set for use with CBM. There are norms for performance and progress, and there are criteria (i.e., benchmarks) that can also be used. These same standards can be used to make two types of decisions within an RTI approach.

The first type of decision is about the effectiveness of the instructional program that a student is receiving. If the student's level of performance or rate of progress is below the standard being used, then the instruction is not as effective as we want it to be. The decision we need to make is about how to alter the instruction the student is receiving in order to increase his level of performance or rate of progress. CBM (or any assessment tool) does not give you information specific enough to determine which instructional approach to use or how to alter the current one—this is the time for teachers, as professionals, to use their professional judgment. No matter how well developed, an assessment tool does not have the same amount of information about the student as a teacher does. There are some structured approaches to decision making (see the Resources and Further Reading section of this chapter for some), but they do not tell you what to do—they only provide guidelines for decision making.

The second type of decision made within RTI is about eligibility for remedial programs such as special education. Most often, this is mentioned in reference to eligibility for the category of Learning Disability (LD), but the decision can also be made for a general determination of eligible/not eligible. This is often referred to as a noncategorical approach to special education since one does not have to determine which disability category a student might belong to before providing services.

The most common method to this approach of eligibility determination is called the *dual discrepancy method*. Because CBM provides you with performance data (the level a student is performing at) and progress data (his rate of growth), you can compare both of these types of data to standards (such as the ones discussed previously in this chapter).

Since this isn't a book on RTI, we really can't go into too much detail. Suffice it to say that CBM is a core component of RTI. If you are interested in learning more about RTI, check out some of the resources listed in the Resources and Further Reading section of this chapter.

COMPUTERIZED GRAPHING AND DATA MANAGEMENT SYSTEMS

There are many different alternatives for computerized graphing and data management programs. Some are designed to be used specifically with the company's products, and others have the flexibility to incorporate other measures as the user wants. All the programs listed below allow the user to enter and graph data. Some are web-based and some are stand-alone programs (meaning you can install them on a single computer or sometimes a local network). Some programs will also allow for data management and storage over time, which enables cross-year analysis and interpretation. Some will even collect and score the data. Cost for the programs varies. For some it depends on the level of license that is purchased (e.g., individual, schoolwide). For others it depends on which services are purchased. There are three general types of computerized systems: material-specific programs, material-flexible programs, and general spreadsheet and data management programs. It is important to select one that is right for your specific needs. Each program is described in terms of the following criteria:

- *Type*: Is the program web-based (meaning that the data are stored on a remote server and are accessed through the Internet) or stand-alone (meaning that the program is installed on a specific computer and must be accessed through that computer)?
- *Data*: Does the program allow for cross-year data management and analysis, or is it only available for within-year use?
- *Fee*: Is there a fee associated with the program or its use? Is it a one-time fee or an ongoing fee for usage?
- *Auto*: Does the program allow for computerized administration and scoring, or is it solely for data management and interpretation?
- *Skills*: Which skills discussed in this book can be addressed using this program?
- *Note*: This provides additional information about the program (if applicable).

Material-Specific Programs

DIBELS Data System (dibels.uoregon.edu)

- *Type*: web-based
- *Data*: cross-year
- *Fee*: ongoing usage fee
- *Auto*: data management and storage
- *Skills*: Reading (ORF only), Early Reading (DIBELS only)
- *Note*: Materials are also available in Spanish.

DIBELS Monitoring Device (DiMonD; e-mail to: cdorman1@cfl.rr.com)

- *Type*: stand-alone
- *Data*: cross-year
- *Fee*: none
- *Auto*: data management and storage
- *Skills*: Reading (ORF only), Early Reading (DIBELS only)

Edcheckup (www.edcheckup.com)

- *Type*: web-based
- *Data*: cross-year
- *Fee*: ongoing usage fee

- *Auto*: computerized scoring (ORF only), data management, and storage
- *Skills*: Reading (ORF, Maze), Early Reading (LSF, WIF), Writing

Yearly Progress Pro (YPP; CTB/McGraw-Hill: *www.ctb.com*)

- *Type*: web-based
- *Data*: cross-year
- *Fee*: ongoing usage fee
- *Auto*: computerized administration, scoring, data management, and storage
- *Skills*: Reading (Maze), Math (Computation, Concepts and Applications)
- *Note*: Math materials do not use the traditional CBM procedures or require a production response.

Material-Flexible Programs

AIMSweb (Pearson; Harcourt Assessment: *www.aimsweb.com*)

- *Type*: web-based
- *Data*: cross-year
- *Fee*: ongoing usage fee
- *Auto*: data management and storage
- *Skills*: Reading, Early Reading (DIBELS, LSF), Spelling, Writing, Math (Early Numeracy, Computation)
- *Note*: Early Reading materials are also available in Spanish. Most skills are linked to AIMSweb-specific materials, but DIBELS measures can also be included.

Intervention Central (Chart Dog: *www.interventioncentral.org*)

- *Type*: web-based
- *Data*: single year
- *Fee*: none
- *Auto*: data management and storage
- *Skills*: Reading, Early Reading (DIBELS, LSF, WIF), Spelling, Writing, Math (Early Numeracy, Computation, Concepts and Applications)
- *Note*: For progress monitoring only. Can be customized to include any CBM measure.

Spreadsheet and Data Management Programs

Excel

- *Type*: stand-alone
- *Data*: cross-year
- *Fee*: one-time fee (comes bundled with Microsoft Office)
- *Auto*: data management and storage
- *Note*: There are some graphs that Excel cannot create; however, data are easily exported into other software that can. Requires more time (due to creating the system from scratch), but is more flexible to meet local needs.

FileMaker Pro

- *Type*: stand-alone (although there is a web-based version)
- *Data*: cross-year
- *Fee*: one-time fee
- *Auto*: data management and storage
- *Note*: Requires more time (due to creating system from scratch), but is more flexible to meet local needs. Not as readily available as Excel (which could create accessibility issues).

FREQUENTLY ASKED QUESTIONS ABOUT CHARTING AND GRAPHING CBM DATA

1. ***Does the use of CBM lead to changes in students' curriculum?*** CBM doesn't lead to changes in curriculum because that is set by state standards or the student's IEP. It does lead to more frequent changes in instruction, and those changes have been shown to lead to increased student performance. Remember, CBM is not a curriculum or an intervention, but it does provide data on how students are responding to a curriculum or intervention.

2. ***Does the median score reliably predict the student's baseline?*** Generally, the median score is considered the baseline. It's not quite the same as in behavior assessment or single-case research, though; it's more like the starting point or a pretreatment score. We can't wait to find a stable baseline over time because we're not measuring skills that should be stable. If a student wasn't improving her performance for 3 or more weeks, we shouldn't be waiting around to try an intervention. We should be panicking.

3. ***If a student reaches his goal early, should I continue to monitor his progress to see if he exceeds the goal?*** Absolutely! You should set a more ambitious goal if the student gets four consecutive scores above his goal line. If the student's goal was to meet a benchmark or catch up to his peers, you could start to monitor his progress less frequently so that you can focus your time on another student having difficulty.

4. *Why is it important to have intervention lines?* Intervention lines are put onto the graph in order for you to be able to separate different interventions or phases of the student's instruction more easily. They let you quickly and clearly tell when something different occurred and judge what effect it might have had on the student's rate of progress.

5. *While progress monitoring a student, how many times do you allow his performance to fall below the goal line before reassessing his instructional level?* When a student's performance falls below the goal line for four consecutive data points, you should consider making an instructional change rather than assuming his instructional level is different. His level of performance is probably fairly stable. It is his rate of progress that is not as good as it should be.

6. *Would it be appropriate to show the student his chart even if his performance is falling below the goal line?* Yes. Students like to see what kind of progress they're making—it can be very motivating when they're doing well and when they're not doing as well as we'd like. Rather than telling the student that he isn't doing well or is failing, the chart can be used to start a discussion about changing instruction (how the discussion goes depends on the student and his grade level). It might start off something like, "You're right. Your progress isn't as good as we want it to be. Maybe we should try something different with how I teach you reading."

7. *When is it appropriate to raise a student's goal?* After collecting a minimum of six to eight data points, a student's goal should be raised when he has four consecutive data points above the goal line.

RESOURCES AND FURTHER READING

Conte, K. L., & Hintze, J. M. (2000). The effects of performance feedback and goal setting on oral reading fluency within curriculum-based measurement. *Diagnostique, 25*(2), 85–98.

Deno, S. L. (1987). Curriculum-based measurement, program development, graphing performance and increasing efficiency. *Teaching Exceptional Children, 20*(1), 41–47.

Howell, K. W., Hosp, J. L., Hosp, M. K., & Macconell, K. (in press). *Curriculum-based evaluation: Linking assessment and instruction.* New York: Sage.

Jimerson, S., Burns, M., & VanDerHeyden, A. (2007). *The handbook of Response to Intervention: The science and practice of assessment and intervention.* New York: Springer.

Marston, D. B., Diment, K., Allen, D., & Allen, L. (1992). Monitoring pupil progress in reading. *Preventing School Failure, 36*(2), 21–25.

National Association of School Psychologists (2006). *Assessment alternatives under IDEA 2004* (CD Rom Toolkit). Bethesda, MD: Author.

Salvia, J., Ysseldyke, J., & Bolt, S. (2007). *Assessment* (10th edition). Boston: Houghton-Mifflin. (Particularly see Chapter 30, "Assessing Response to Intervention")

9

Planning to Use CBM—
and Keeping It Going

Our best intentions will not go far without a solid plan for carrying them out. It is worth putting in the time and effort up front to ensure successful implementing of CBM. Getting it going is only half of it, though; planning how to keep it going is the other half and just as important. In this chapter, we outline ways to help plan for using CBM before, during, and after initial implementation. We also offer helpful hints on how to get and keep CBM going.

DEVELOPING A PLAN FOR USING CBM

So you have decided to implement CBM. Congratulations! With a well-developed plan you will soon see how CBM will allow you to help all students achieve greater success in school. This is possible because CBM provides a database for each student which allows you to evaluate the effectiveness of the instruction they are receiving. Whether you are looking at implementing CBM at the classroom, grade, schoolwide, or district level, the factors that need to be considered will be similar.

We have broken the task of planning to use CBM into 10 steps. In Appendix B we provide a checklist to get you started. Below are points to consider to ensure you are making informed decisions as you complete the checklist.

Ten Steps to Using CBM before, during, and after Initial Implementation

Before

STEP 1: WHO WILL BE USING CBM?

This depends on what it will be used for. Below each group are some points to consider.

- *Classroom(s)*: Is this something only one teacher is interested in? If yes, then this teacher will be able to screen/benchmark and track the progress of her class, but she will not be able to compare how her students are doing to others in the school or district.
- *Grade(s)*: Is this something only one grade is interested in? If yes, the teachers in that grade will be able to screen/benchmark and track progress for all of their students but, they will not be able to compare how their students are doing to others in that school or district.
- *School(s)*: Is this something only one school is interested in? If yes, teachers in that school will be able to screen/benchmark and track progress for all of their students. This will help them track students from year to year and will provide a good overall indication of how the students are achieving in the school, but if only one or two schools use CBM, then they will not be able to compare how their students are doing to others in the district.
- *District*: Is the district deciding to adopt CBM for every school? If yes, teachers in that district will be able to screen/benchmark and track progress of every student enrolled. They will also be able to track progress even if students move from one school to another, but if every school decides to use a different program or set of materials, then the data may not be comparable across schools.

STEP 2: WHICH CBM SKILLS WILL BE IMPLEMENTED?

This may be a hard question to answer if you are interested in all of the areas of CBM. Since the majority of student problems in school are in the area of reading, it might be a good place to start. Below each area are some points to consider.

- *Early reading* (LSF, WIF, DIBELS): Skill level of students is important to consider—some early reading skills are not needed for students who have already mastered them.
- *Reading* (ORF, Mazes): Only Mazes can be administered to a group, but reading is a critical area, and these measures are great for screening/benchmarking and progress monitoring.
- *Spelling* (CLS, WSC): Can be administered to a group, which saves time.
- *Writing* (TWW, WSC, CWS): Is the longest CBM measure to implement, but can be administered to a group, which saves time. It would be a great add-on once one of the other areas is going strong.
- *Math* (Early Numeracy, Computation, Concepts and Applications): Can be administered to a group, which saves time.

STEP 3: WHAT MATERIALS WILL WE USE?

This is a very important decision that will make the process either easy or hard. Below each area are some points to consider.

- *Commercial product with graphing program*: These can be a real time saver as well as offering some of the better products out there. These programs are usually web-based, meaning that the data can be entered and viewed from anywhere. The data can be looked at by the individual student, teachers, principals, and other administrators. In some cases, parents can get online access to their child(ren)'s data.
- *Purchase premade material and make your own graphing program*: This option is probably best if just one or two teachers are going to be using CBM. The downside is that you have to photocopy and organize the material as well as build and run your own graphing program. Sources for obtaining premade material are provided in text boxes in each of the content chapters.
- *Purchase premade material and graph on paper*: This option is probably only reasonable for the single teacher who will be using CBM only for her class or for a few students.

STEP 4: WHEN WILL IMPLEMENTATION START?

Timing is everything, so it is important to plan as far ahead as possible. One thing to remember is that you will need a few weeks to prepare for training, ordering and getting the materials together, and practicing. Below each area are some points to consider.

- *Fall*: This is the best time to start with screening/benchmarking and progress monitoring. This will mean planning at the end of the previous year or over the summer before students arrive.
- *Winter*: If training, materials, and organization don't come together in the fall, then waiting until winter may be a better plan than rushing only to have it done incorrectly. You can still screen/benchmark all students and start progress monitoring in the winter; you will just not have the benefit of the fall data for this first year.
- *Spring*: This is the last choice for when to start; however, it could be used to introduce staff to CBM, conduct some training, and practice giving the measures. If you use this model, you will want to make sure that a review training is also included in the fall since there will be a period of time during which staff will not have used the measures.

STEP 5: WHO WILL TRAIN THE STAFF?

The message sometimes is only as good as the messenger. We have seen the best of practices implemented poorly due to poor training. It is usually worth the money to make sure the training is done well and at the level of sophistication that the staff needs. Below each area are some points to consider.

• Hire a professional trainer to train the staff: Not all professional training is equal, so ask around and try to use people who have expertise and can provide excellent training. If resources are an issue, then try to coordinate these efforts with other schools and possibly other districts nearby. Good training can make all the difference. Along these lines, follow-up training should also be built into the plan. Having someone come back and help troubleshoot as well as assist with interpreting the data is well worth it.

• Have a couple of staff members receive professional training and then train the rest of the staff: This can save time and expense and work well if the staff members being trained already have a strong knowledge base in CBM. If not, the information shared may not be a true representation of how to conduct CBM.

• Train yourselves by using published materials and practicing together as a group: If professional training is not an option, then getting a group together to learn and practice the materials may be the way to go. One caution is that the group should already have some knowledge of assessment and understand the importance of standardized directions. More time to learn and practice will need to be built into this model so that when CBM is conducted it is done correctly.

During

STEP 6: WHO WILL MANAGE THE MATERIALS?

This is an organization and time-management issue. Managing the materials can include purchasing, printing and collating, distributing, storing, and putting student names on materials. The person responsible for managing the material needs to have time allocated for this task. It takes time to purchase or print material and organize it for every teacher and student. It is best to organize the material well in advance so that things can be double-checked. This also allows for time to practice administering and scoring the measures prior to collecting data. Below each area are some points to consider.

• *Teacher* (general education, Title I, ESL, special education): Having an individual teacher manage the materials can be a smart way to go since teachers are already familiar with the details that go into testing students. They are often better at thinking up strategies to improve the efficiency of making, collecting, and storing materials.

• *Administrator* (prinicipal, vice principal): Having an administrator manage the materials is a nice way to involve him or her in the process but most administrators have schedules that prohibit them from managing the materials on a day-to-day basis. It might be better to include administrators in the training and possibly in the collection of data.

• *Support staff* (speech therapist, reading specialist, school psychologist): Having support staff manage the materials can be a good way to get them involved and working directly with the other educators in the school. One problem is that support staff may not always be in your building, making it hard to reach them at times.

• *Assistant* (administrative assistants, parent volunteers): Having an administrative assistant or parent volunteer may be a good choice if they have the time and organizational skills. With any volunteer, you want to be careful about confidentiality issues related to students' work.

STEP 7: WHO WILL COLLECT THE DATA?

This is critical to the time it will take to collect the data as well as who has ownership of it. Time and ownership of the data are the two main issues that should guide you when making a plan. In addition, making sure the data are collected with fidelity is critical. See the General Fidelity Checklist for Conducting CBM in Appendix B to assist with this. Below each area are some points to consider.

• *Individual teachers*: Having teachers help with data collection allows them to learn CBM and have an understanding of the tasks, what the student is asked to perform, and what the results mean. Our experience has been that if teachers do not collect the data for their own students, they may view them as "your data" and not "their data." When it comes to progress monitoring, teachers should collect the data for their own students. When screening/benchmarking, it may be more efficient to have a team where the teacher helps collect some of the data in her class but is not responsible for the collection of all the data.

• *Teams* (general and special education teachers, educational assistants, principals, school psychologists, reading specialists, speech therapists): This is a great approach to use when collecting data for screening/benchmarking. The more people at the school or district who are trained, the faster the data collection will go. It also shows that people value what is happening enough to get involved and help out. This is especially true if the principal joins in. A word of caution about using parent volunteers and older students to help collect the data. We have found that confidentiality can be jeopardized by including people who are not directly employed by the school. Parents and older students also often do not have the expertise in assessment to ensure the data are collected correctly.

STEP 8: WHERE WILL THE DATA BE COLLECTED?

This is also a time-management issue. It should be done in the most efficient way that will provide the least amount of disruption to teaching while collecting the data quickly.

• *In the classroom*: This can be done by having the individual teacher assess all of her own students. This takes time away from teaching, however, and may not be the fastest way to collect the data. A team could go into the classroom and help assess all of the students. While this may not take as much time away from teaching, it may not be the fastest way to collect the data because the team would have to organize each classroom separately as well as bring all of the materials with them.

• *Central location* (library, cafeteria, multipurpose room): This takes little time away from teaching and is the best way to collect all the data quickly. A team would only have to organize one room as they would have all of their material in one place and could move through classrooms of students rather quickly. One way to speed this process up is to have classrooms come to the central location as a group. While some students are being assessed, others can be kept busy by reading a book silently while being supervised. This is where parent volunteers and other staff can help out by supervising those students waiting and bringing in the next class when the team is ready.

After

STEP 9: WHO WILL MANAGE THE DATA ONCE THEY ARE COLLECTED?

There are simple ways to manage the data that will make using CBM time and energy efficient. This step, like all of the others, is critical to the success of using any type of assessment. Below each area are some points to consider.

- *Each teacher is responsible for entering and graphing her students' data*: This is not a bad idea if this time can be planned for and built into teachers' schedules. It would allow for a quick turnaround time from when students were assessed to when graphs are printed. It is not necessarily the task of entering and graphing that makes the difference, however, but rather the act of looking at the data and planning instruction. Therefore, it is not always necessary for teachers to do this.
- *One person for each grade or school is responsible for entering and graphing the data*: This may be more time efficient if there are people at each school who could have this task built into their duties. This would mean that they would have to have times where they would be available to enter the data and print graphs. Having one or more people to do this assigned at each school may decrease the turnaround time from when the students were assessed to when the data are entered and graphs printed.
- *A team of people at the district is responsible for entering and graphing the data*: Having someone at the district level to perform this task would be the last resort. If the data need to be moved to another location to be entered and then the graphs had to be brought back to each school, this could increase the lag between assessing the students and getting the information back. It is not a bad idea, however, to have someone at the district level who understands the assessment and can assist in reading and interpreting the data.

STEP 10: HOW WILL THE DATA BE SHARED?

If the data are collected, entered, graphed, and printed but then put into a drawer, they may as well not have been collected at all. A wise principal once told us "Out of sight is out of mind. I want my teachers looking at their data every day." This last step closes the circle and makes the process whole. Below each area are some points to consider.

- *Each teacher is responsible for looking at her data by herself*: If only one teacher in the school is using CBM, then this would be OK, but it is more efficient and effective to have teachers working together to determine what the data mean as well as identifying interventions to use.

- *At the grade level, all of the teachers look at all of the students together*: This is a great way for the teachers in each grade to look at individual students as well as identify groups of students that may need additional help. A team approach is always preferred over a single person when looking at the data.

- *At the school level, a team is responsible for looking at all of the students*: This may be time efficient, but if the team members are not familiar with the students, they may have a harder time understanding what to do about individual students. Looking at the grade levels to identify trends and possible areas of weakness in the curriculum would be appropriate at this level.

HINTS ON HOW TO GET CBM GOING

There are many ways to approach getting CBM going in a classroom, grade, school, or district. The most effective way is to have a team of people, including someone from the administration, such as a principal, a district coordinator for assessment or special services, or even a superintendent. Other members could be general education or special education teachers and specialists like reading coaches, speech therapists, school psychologists, or counselors. We have found the implementation and sustainability to be greater with a group of people working together for a common goal.

This team can educate others on some of the reasons to use CBM. The following lists provide some ideas and pointers to use.

- It is fast and efficient to give and score.
- It provides excellent information on students' overall skills in reading, spelling, writing, and math.
- It is fluency based.
- It allows for more time teaching and less time assessing.
- It can be used to group students and help plan instruction.
- It can be used to screen/benchmark all students at least three times per year.
- It allows for monitoring progress throughout the year in an easy and quick manner.
- It is a reliable and valid measure of students' skills that has more than 25 years of research behind it.
- It could replace other more costly and lengthy tests.

HINTS ON HOW TO KEEP CBM GOING

Planning ahead and being prepared for questions is one way to ensure that CBM will become a standard in a school or district. It will take work to keep it going. Below we provide a list of activities and ideas to help.

- Prepare the materials ahead of time for the entire year. This would include materials needed to screen/benchmark and progress monitor. Some tips are to color-code student books by grades so that they are easy to identify when testing multiple grades. Having the students' names printed on labels and placed on the materials can also save a lot of time. Make extra copies of student materials for retesting or in case students move into the district. Another tip is to have the teacher/examiner materials laminated or put in pocket protectors and into a binder so that they are easy to locate and will have sustainability over the years.

- Have a schedule planned before the year starts. Putting dates down on a calendar for the entire year will help everyone plan when screening/benchmarking will occur, when progress monitoring will happen, and when graphs will be printed. Reminding everyone of what is happening can easily be done by distributing a monthly calendar (or adding these things to the school monthly calendar that is already developed) with the CBM information specific to that month. One tip is to wait at least 2 instructional weeks before conducting any assessments (especially screening/benchmarks). Some students need time after a break to get back in the swing of things, and if we assess them too early, they will not have the opportunity to show us their best skills.

- Incorporating the data into everyday use. The data could be brought to weekly grade-level meetings, and any students who are struggling could be discussed. Another way to incorporate the data is to send home weekly progress-monitoring sheets to parents so they can see how their children are doing. This information could also be shared at parent–teacher conferences. The scores could be incorporated on the students' report cards.

- Regularly share successes with colleagues. This could take place at weekly or monthly staff or grade-level meetings. A more formal way to do this would be to put out a newsletter that highlights the successes of CBM throughout the district or school.

- Conduct follow-up or review sessions when needed. Especially during the first year, it will be helpful to have review sessions that allow staff to ask questions now that they are becoming more familiar with the assessment procedures. It might be helpful to hire a consultant to assist with this if there is currently no one on staff who is qualified or experienced enough to answer these questions.

- Rotate the person in charge of managing the collection of the data so that she does not get burned out. This will also give others an opportunity to learn additional skills when collecting and using CBM data. One suggestion would be to rotate it from grade to grade each quarter, half year, or year.

FREQUENTLY ASKED QUESTIONS ABOUT PLANNING AND USING CBM

1. *As a special educator, will I be allowed to use CBM if the school doesn't use it?* Yes. If you write your IEP goals and objectives using CBM data, you will not only be allowed to use it but required to. Special educators need to monitor all of their students

closely. CBM allows you to do this in a timely and efficient manner so that you can determine which students are responding to your instruction and which are not.

2. *How can I persuade my school to adopt CBM or at least allow me to use it?* None of us has met an administrator who has said "no" when asked, "If I can track students' progress every week using an assessment that is reliable and valid and will only take me 3–5 minutes per student, would you say 'yes'?" Another way to sell it is to show the administrator the graphs and how you will track progress toward goals that will inform you, the student, the administrator, and the parents.

3. *Can anyone administer CBM assessments? Can a paraprofessional give them?* There are people we would recommend and not recommend for administering CBM assessments; however, anyone who works at a school should be able to be trained and supervised so that they can help collect CBM data. People we do not recommend using are parent volunteers and students due to confidentiality issues and reliability in administering and scoring the assessments.

4. *Would it be a good idea to involve the parents of a struggling student to also conduct CBM at home, or should it only be done in the classroom?* The data collection should only be conducted by one person to ensure the reliability and accuracy of the data collected. Therefore, we would recommend having only the teacher administer CBM. It is a great idea to involve parents by sending home the student graphs on a weekly basis and encouraging parents to have their children read aloud to them. If you also want the parent to collect CBM data, you should provide them with their own CBM graph to use while you keep yours at school.

RESOURCES AND FURTHER READING

Allinder, R. M. (1996). When some is not better than none: Effects of differential implementation of curriculum-based measurement. *Exceptional Children, 62,* 525–535.

Allinder, R. M., & BeckBest, M. A. (1995). Differential effects of two approaches to supporting teachers' use of curriculum-based measurement. *School Psychology Review, 24,* 287–298.

Burns, M. K. (2002). Comprehensive system of assessment to intervention using curriculum-based assessments. *Intervention in School and Clinic, 38*(1), 8–13.

Fuchs, L. S., & Fuchs, D. (1993). Effects of systematic observation and feedback on teachers' implementation of curriculum-based measurement. *Teacher Education and Special Education, 16,* 178–187.

Hasbrouck, J. E., Woldbeck, T., Ihnot, C., & Parker, R. I. (1999). One teacher's use of curriculum-based measurement: A changed opinion. *Learning Disabilities Research and Practice, 14,* 118–126.

Howe, K. B., Scierka, B. J., Gibbons, K. A., & Silberglitt, B. (2003). A schoolwide organization system for raising reading achievement using general outcome measures and evidence-based instruction: One education district's experience. *Assessment for Effective Intervention, 28*(3/4), 59–71.

Marston, D. B., & Magnusson, D. (1985). Implementing curriculum-based measurement in special and regular education settings. *Exceptional Children, 52,* 266–276.

Whinnery, K. W., & Fuchs, L. S. (1992). Implementing effective teaching strategies with learning disabled students through curriculum-based measurement. *Learning Disabilities Research and Practice, 7*(1), 25–30.

Yell, M. L., Deno, S. L., & Marston, D. B. (1992). Barriers to implementing curriculum-based measurement. *Diagnostique, 18*(1), 99–112.

Appendix A

Summary of Validity and Reliability Studies for CBM

Here is a summary of the validity and reliability studies conducted on all areas of CBM. Because there are literally hundreds of studies, we have chosen to highlight only three recent studies in each area. For a more complete review of the studies in each area, see AIMSweb (2006), Good and Jefferson (1998), and Marston (1989).

VALIDITY STUDIES

Skill area	Study	Subjects	Criterion measure	Correlations
Reading (WRC)	Jenkins, Fuchs, et al. (2000)	113; grade 4	Iowa Test of Basic Skills (ITBS)	.83
Reading (WRC)	Hintze, Shapiro, Conte, & Basile (1997)	57; grades 2–4	Degrees of Reading Power Test (DRP)	.66
Reading (WRC)	Madelaine & Wheldall (1998)	50; grades 1–5	Neale Analysis of Reading—Revised	.71
Spelling (WSC and CLS)	Marston (1982)	37; grades 4–6	Stanford Achievement Spelling subtest	.87 (WSC) .81 (CLS)
Spelling (WSC and CLS)	Deno, Mirkin, Lowry, & Kuehnle (1980)	45; grades 2–6	Peabody Individual Achievement Tests	.88 (WSC) .81 (CLS)
Spelling (WSC and CLS)	Deno, Mirkin, Lowry, & Kuehnle (1980)	42; grades 2–6	Test of Written Spelling	.95 (WSC) .98 (CLS)
Writing (TWW, WSC, and CWS)	Fewster & MacMillan (2002)	465; grades 6–7	School grade in grades 8–10	.31–.50 (WSC)
Writing (TWW, WSC, and CWS)	Espin, Shin, Deno, Skare, Robinson, & Benner (2000)	121; grades 7–8	District Writing Test	.43–.47 (TWW) .46–.51 (WSC) .61–.65 (CWS)
Writing (TWW, WSC, and CWS)	Espin, Scierka, Skare, & Halverson (1999)	147; grade 10	California Achievement Test—Language Arts Total	.13 (TWW) .17 (WSC) .29 (CWS)

141

Skill area	Study	Subjects	Criterion measure	Correlations
Math (CD)	Thurber & Shinn (2002)	207; grade 4	Stanford Diagnostic Math Computation; California Achievement Test Computation; Latent Construct of Math Computation	.58 .62 .64
Math (CD)	Skiba et al. (1986)	58; grades 5–6	MAT Problem Solving; District CRT Basic Math Concepts	.52 and .67 (5th grade) .65 and .58 (6th grade)
Math (CD)	Skiba et al. (1986)	65; grades 3–4	MAT Problem Solving; District CRT Basic Math Concepts	.37 and .29 (3rd grade) .45 and .37 (4th grade)

RELIABILITY STUDIES

Skill area	Study	Subjects	Type of reliability	Correlations
Reading (WRC)	Tindal, Germann, et al. (1983)	110; grade 4	Two parallel forms at same time	.94
Reading (WRC)	Marston (1982)	83; grades 3–6	Test–retest (1 week apart) Test–retest (10 weeks apart)	.90 .82
Reading (WRC)	Shinn (1981)	71; grade 5	Test–retest (5 weeks apart)	.90
Spelling (WSC and CLS)	Tindal, Germann, et al. (1988)	566; grades 1–6	Test–retest (20 weeks apart) Two parallel forms at same time Interjudge scoring	.91, .96, .99 (WSC) .86, .97., .91 (CLS)
Spelling (WSC and CLS)	Marston (1982)	83; grades 3–6	Test–retest (10 weeks apart)	.87 (WSC) .92 (CLS)
Spelling (WSC and CLS)	Shinn (1981)	71; grade 5	Test–retest (5 weeks apart)	.85 (WSC) .83 (CLS)
Writing (TWW, WSC, and CWS)	Maleki & Jewell (2003)	946; grades 1–6	Interscorer agreement	> 99% (TWW) > 99% (WSC) > 98% (CWS)
Writing (TWW, WSC, and CWS)	Gansle, Noell, VanDerHeyden, Naquin, & Slider (2002)	179; grades 3–4	Interscorer agreement and Alternate Form	96% (TWW) 95% (WSC) 86% (CWS) .62 (TWW) .53 (WSC) .46 (CWS)
Writing (TWW, WSC, and CWS)	Espin, Shin, Deno, Skare, Robinson, & Benner (2000)	147; grade 10	Interscorer agreement	100% (TWW) 99.5% (WSC) 97.4% (CWS)
Math (CD)	Thurber & Shinn (2002)	207; grade 4	Interscorer agreement and Alternate Form	.83 .91
Math (CD)	Fuchs, Fuchs, & Hamlett (1989)	62; grades 3–9	Internal consistency and interscorer agreement	.93 .93
Math (CD)	Tindal, Germann, et al. (1983)	30; grade 5	Test–retest (1 week apart)	.93

Appendix B

Reproducible Quick Guides and Forms for Conducting CBM

CHAPTER 3

Quick Administration Guide for ORF CBM   145

Quick Scoring Guide for ORF CBM   146

Quick Administration Guide for Maze CBM with Practice Items   147

Quick Administration Guide for Maze CBM without Practice Items   148

Survey-Level Assessment for ORF   149

CHAPTER 4

Quick Administration Guide for LSF CBM   150

Quick Scoring Guide for LSF CBM   150

Quick Administration Guide for WIF CBM   151

Quick Scoring Guide for WIF CBM   151

CHAPTER 5

Quick Administration Guide for Spelling CBM (Grades 1 and 2)   152

Quick Administration Guide for Spelling CBM (Grades 3+)   152

Quick Scoring Guide for Spelling CBM   153

CHAPTER 6

Quick Administration Guide for Writing CBM   154

Quick Scoring Guide for Writing CBM (WSC)   154

Quick Scoring Guide for Writing CBM (CWS)   155

CHAPTER 7

Quick Administration Guide for Math CBM (mixed-math)   156

Quick Administration Guide for Math CBM (single-skill)   156

Quick Scoring Guide for Math CBM   157

Survey-Level Assessment for Math   158

CHAPTER 8

Graph for Progress-Monitoring Data   159

CHAPTER 9

Checklist for Using CBM before, during, and after Initial Implementation   160

General Fidelity Checklist for Conducting CBM   162

QUICK ADMINISTRATION GUIDE FOR ORF CBM

1. Place the copy of the student passage in front of the student.
2. Place the teacher/examiner copy on the clipboard so the student cannot see it.
3. Say: *"When I say 'Begin,' start reading aloud at the top of the page. Read across the page* (point to the first line of the passage). *Try to read each word. If you come to a word you don't know, I'll tell it to you. Be sure to do your best reading. Do you have any questions? Begin."* (*Trigger stopwatch or timer for 1 minute.*)
4. Follow along on the teacher/examiner copy as the student reads and put a slash (/) through any incorrect words.
5. At the end of 1 minute, say: *"Thank you"* and mark the last word read with a bracket (]).

Adapted from Shinn (1989)

QUICK ADMINISTRATION GUIDE FOR ORF CBM

1. Place the copy of the student passage in front of the student.
2. Place the teacher/examiner copy on the clipboard so the student cannot see it.
3. *"I would like you to read this story aloud for me. Please start here* (point to the first word on the student's copy) *and read aloud. This is not a race. Try each word. If you come to a word that you do not know, you may skip it and go to the next word. You may start when I say 'Begin.' You may stop when I say 'Stop reading.' Do you have any questions? Begin."* (*Trigger stopwatch or timer for 1 minute.*)
4. Follow along on the teacher/examiner copy as the student reads and put an X through any incorrect words.
5. At the end of 1 minute, say *"Stop reading"* and mark the end of the last word read with a slash (/).

Adapted from Edcheckup (2005)

QUICK SCORING GUIDE FOR ORF CBM

Scored as Correct

- A word must be pronounced correctly, in accordance with the context of the sentence.

- Repetitions: Words said over again are ignored.

- Self-corrections: Words misread initially but corrected within 3 seconds are scored as correct.

- Insertions: If the student adds extra words, those words are counted neither as correct nor as errors.

- Dialect/articulation: Variations in pronunciation explainable by local language norms or speech sound production are correct.

(continued on other side)

Scored as Errors

- Mispronunciations/word substitutions: Words either mispronounced or substituted with other words are errors.

- Omissions: Each word omitted is an error.

- Hesitations: When a student hesitates to pronounce a word correctly within **3 seconds**, the student is told the word and an error is scored.

- Reversals: When a student transposes two or more words, those words not read in the correct order are errors.

Special Scoring Examples

- Numerals: Numbers are counted as words and must be read correctly within the context of the passage.

- Hyphenated words: Each morpheme separated by a hyphen(s) is counted as an individual word if it can stand alone.

- Abbreviations: Abbreviations are counted as words and must be read correctly within the context of the sentence (e.g., Mrs., Dr.).

QUICK ADMINISTRATION GUIDE FOR MAZE CBM WITH PRACTICE ITEMS

1. Place a copy of the student passage with the *practice items* in front of each student.

2. Say: ***"Today I want you to read a short story. The story you will read has some places where you will need to choose the correct word. Read the story. When you come to three words in dark print, choose the word that belongs in the sentence.***

    "We will do some examples. Look at the first page. Read the sentence. The sentence says: 'Bill threw the ball to Jane. Jane caught the (dog, bat, ball).' Which one of the three words belongs in the sentence?"

3. After the students respond, say: ***"The word** ball **belongs in the sentence 'Bill threw the ball to Jane. Jane caught the ball.' Circle the word** ball."***

4. ***"Now let's try sentence number two. Read the sentence. The sentence says: Tom said, "Now you (jump, throw, talk) the ball to me.' Which of the three words belongs in the sentence?"***

5. After the students respond say: ***"The word** throw **belongs in the sentence 'Now you throw the ball to me.' Circle the word** throw."***

6. Place a copy of the student passage in front of each student face down.

(continued on other side)

---

7. Say: ***"Now you are going to do the same thing by yourself. You will read a story for 1 minute. When I say 'Stop,' stop reading. Do not begin reading until I tell you to start. Whenever you come to three words that are in dark print, circle the word that belongs in the sentence.***

    "Choose a word even if you're not sure of the answer. At the end of 1 minute, I will say 'Stop.' If you finish early, check your answers. Do not go on to the next page. You may turn your paper over and begin when I say Start. Are there any questions?

    "Remember to do the best you can. Pick up your pencils. Ready? Start."
   (Trigger stop watch or timer for 1 minute.)

8. Walk around the room to monitor that students are only circling one word per set and not skipping around the page.

9. At the end of 1 minute, say: ***"Stop. Put your pencils down."***

10. Separately administer two more passages using the following directions.

11. Say: ***"Now you will do the same thing with another story. Remember to choose the word that belongs in the sentence. Choose a word even if you're not sure of the answer. You may begin when I tell you to."*** *(Trigger stopwatch or timer for 1 minute.)*

12. At the end of 1 minute, say: ***"Stop. Put your pencils down."***

13. Collect all the student sheets.

Adapted from Edcheckup (2005)

QUICK ADMINISTRATION GUIDE FOR MAZE CBM WITHOUT PRACTICE ITEMS

1. Place a copy of the student passage in front of each student face down. (It is helpful to have the student's name already on the sheet before starting.)

2. Say: *"When I say 'Begin,' turn to the first story and start reading silently. When you come to a group of three words, circle the one word that makes the most sense. Work as quickly as you can without making mistakes. If you finish the page, turn the page and keep working until I say 'Stop' or you are all done. Do you have any questions? Begin."* (Trigger stopwatch or timer for 3 minutes.)

3. Walk around the room to monitor that students are only circling one word per set and not skipping around the page.

4. At the end of 3 minutes say, **"Stop. Put your pencil down and turn your sheet over."**

5. Collect all the student sheets.

Adapted from AIMSweb (2002)

SURVEY-LEVEL ASSESSMENT FOR ORF

Student: _____ **Grade:** _____ **Date:** _____

Examiner: _____

Directions: Starting at the student's grade level, select three passages. Have the student read each orally for one minute. Record the words read correctly (WRC) and number of errors. Continue testing down in reading levels until the student is able to successfully meet the performance criteria (see below).

For each reading level assessed, use the table below to record the following:

- Reading level of passage (e.g., 2)
- Number of errors
- Number of words read correctly (i.e., total words read minus errors)

- Median WRC (middle score of 3)
- Median errors (middle score of 3)

TABLE OF SCORES

READING LEVEL	PASSAGE #1 WRC/ERRORS	PASSAGE #2 WRC/ERRORS	PASSAGE #3 WRC/ERRORS	MEDIAN WRC/ERRORS
	/	/	/	/
	/	/	/	/
	/	/	/	/
	/	/	/	/

CRITERIA FOR DETERMINING STUDENT'S INSTRUCTIONAL LEVEL

INSTRUCTIONAL LEVEL	WORDS READ CORRECTLY (EXPECTED RANGE)	READING ERRORS (EXPECTED RANGE)
1–2	40–60	4 or fewer
3–6	70–100	6 or fewer

STUDENT PERFORMANCE GRAPH

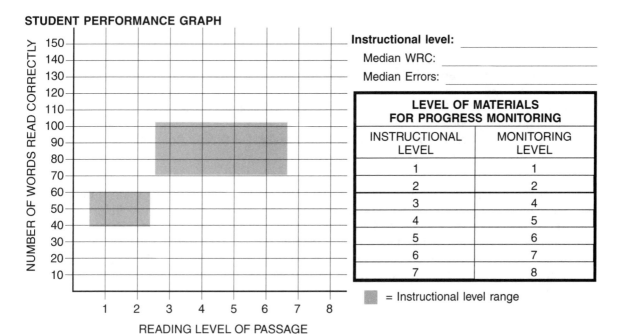

Instructional level: _____

Median WRC: _____

Median Errors: _____

LEVEL OF MATERIALS FOR PROGRESS MONITORING	
INSTRUCTIONAL LEVEL	MONITORING LEVEL
1	1
2	2
3	4
4	5
5	6
6	7
7	8

▓ = Instructional level range

QUICK ADMINISTRATION GUIDE FOR LSF CBM

1. Place the copy of the student sheet in front of the student.

2. Place the teacher/examiner copy on the clipboard so the student cannot see it.

3. Say: *"**Here are some letters** (point to the student copy). **Begin here** (point to the first letter) **and tell me the SOUNDS of as many letters as you can. If you come to a letter you don't know, I'll tell it to you. Are there any questions? Put your finger under the first letter. Ready? Begin.**" (Trigger stopwatch or timer for 1 minute.)*

4. Follow along on the teacher/examiner copy as the student reads and put a slash (/) through any incorrect letters.

5. At the end of 1 minute say: *"**Thank you**"* and put a bracket (]) after the last sound provided.

Adapted from AIMSweb (2002)

QUICK SCORING GUIDE FOR LSF CBM

Scored as Correct
- A letter sound must be pronounced correctly, using the most common sound.
- Short vowel (not long vowel) sounds are considered correct.
- Self-corrections: Sounds mispronounced initially but corrected within 3 seconds are scored as correct and "sc" is written above the letter.
- Dialect/articulation: Variations in pronunciation explainable by local language norms or speech sound production are correct.
- Added vowel or schwa sound: Sounds with the added "uh" sound are considered correct.

Scored as Errors
- Mispronunciations/letter sound substitutions: Letter sounds either mispronounced or substituted with other letter sounds are errors.
- Omissions: Each letter sound omitted is an error.
- Hesitations: When a student hesitates to pronounce the sound correctly within **3 seconds**, the student is told the sound and an error is scored.
- Reversals: When a student transposes two or more sounds, those sounds not read in the correct order are errors.

QUICK ADMINISTRATION GUIDE FOR WIF CBM

1. Place the copy of the student list in front of the student.

2. Place the teacher/examiner copy on the clipboard so the student cannot see it.

3. Say: *"When I say, 'Begin,' I want you to read these words as quickly and correctly as you can. Start here* (point to the first word) *and go down the page* (run your finger down the first column). *If you don't know a word, skip it and try the next word. Keep reading until I say 'Stop.' Do you have any questions? Begin."*(Trigger stopwatch or timer for 1 minute.)

4. Follow along on the teacher/examiner copy as the student reads and *put a slash (/) through any incorrect words.*

5. At the end of 1 minute, say: *"Stop"* and put a bracket (]) after the last word read.

Adapted from Fuchs and Fuchs (2004)

QUICK SCORING GUIDE FOR WIF CBM

Scored as Correct

- A word must be pronounced correctly to be scored as correct.
- Self-corrections: Words mispronounced initially but corrected within 3 seconds are scored as correct.
- Dialect/articulation: Variations in pronunciation explainable by local language norms or speech sound production are correct.

Scored as Errors

- Mispronunciations/word substitutions: Words either mispronounced or substituted with other words are errors.
- Omissions: Each word omitted is an error.
- Hesitations with no attempt to read word: When a student hesitates for **2 seconds**, the student is prompted to read the next word by pointing to it and saying **"What word?"**
- Hesitations when sounding out a word: When a student is sounding out a word for **5 seconds**, the student is prompted to read the next word by pointing to the next word and saying **"What word?"**
- Reversals: When a student transposes two or more words, those words not read in the correct order are errors.

QUICK ADMINISTRATION GUIDE FOR SPELLING CBM (GRADES 1 AND 2)

1. Select an appropriate grade-level spelling list.
2. Have students number their papers 1 to 12.
3. Say: *"I am going to read some words to you. I want you to write the words on the sheet in front of you. Write the first word on the first line, the second word on the second line, and so on. I'll give you 10 seconds to spell each word. When I say the next word, try to write it, even if you haven't finished the last one. Are there any questions?"*
4. Say the first word and trigger stopwatch or timer for 2 minutes.
5. Say each word twice. Use homonyms in a sentence.
6. Say a new word every 10 seconds.
7. At the end of 2 minutes, say: *"Thank you. Put your pencils down."*

Adapted from Shinn (1989)

QUICK ADMINISTRATION GUIDE FOR SPELLING CBM (GRADES 3+)

1. Select an appropriate grade-level spelling list.
2. Have students number their papers 1 to 17.
3. Say: *"I am going to read some words to you. I want you to write the words on the sheet in front of you. Write the first word on the first line, the second word on the second line, and so on. I'll give you 7 seconds to spell each word. When I say the next word, try to write it, even if you haven't finished the last one. Are there any questions?"*
4. Say the first word and trigger stopwatch or timer for 2 minutes.
5, Say each word twice. Use homonyms in a sentence.
6. Say a new word every 7 seconds.
7. At the end of 2 minutes, say: *"Thank you. Put your pencils down."*

Adapted from Shinn (1989)

QUICK SCORING GUIDE FOR SPELLING CBM

Scored as Correct

- CLS is the number of correct sequences related to spelling, the space before and after the word, and the letter to punctuation (before and after).
- When scoring CLS, the scorer places a caret (^) to indicate each correct sequence.
- Compound words: Words need to stay together without a space.
- Apostrophe: The spaces before and after an apostrophe are counted.
- Hyphens: The spaces before and after a hyphen are counted.
- Capitalization: A word that should be capitalized must begin with a capital letter.
- Repeated letters in sequence: Words with letters that are repeated in sequence are scored the same as If each letter were different.
- Additional letters: Additional letters are not counted twice.
- Insertions: Extra letters at the beginning and end are not counted.

QUICK ADMINISTRATION GUIDE FOR WRITING CBM

1. Provide students with a pencil and piece of lined paper or writing notebook.
2. Select an appropriate story starter.
3. Say: "**Today I want you to write a story. I am going to read a sentence to you first and then I want you to compose a short story about what happens. You will have 1 minute to think about what you will write and 3 minutes to write your story. Remember to do your best work. If you do not know how to spell a word, you should guess. Are there any questions?** (*Pause*) **Put your pencils down and listen. For the next minute, think about** . . . (*insert story starter*)."
4. After reading the story starter, begin your stopwatch and allow *1 minute* for the student(s) to think. (Monitor students so that they do not begin writing.) After *30 seconds* say: "**You should be thinking about** . . . (*insert story starter*)." At the end of *1 minute*, restart your stopwatch for 3 minutes and say: "**Now begin writing.**"
5. Monitor students' attention to the task. Encourage the students to work if they are not writing.
6. After *90 seconds* say: "**You should be writing about** . . . (*insert story starter*)."
7. At the end of *3 minutes* say: "**Thank you. Put your pencils down.**"

Adapted from AIMSweb (2004)

QUICK SCORING GUIDE FOR WRITING CBM (WSC)

Scored as Correct

- Words spelled correctly (WSC) is the number of correctly spelled words, regardless of context in which they are used. Words are counted in WSC if they can be found in the English language. Incorrectly spelled words should be circled.
- WSC is calculated by subtracting the total number of circled words from the total words within.
- Abbreviations: Common abbreviations must be spelled correctly.
- Hyphenated words: Each morpheme counted as an individual word must be spelled correctly. If the morpheme cannot stand alone (e.g., prefix) and part of the word is incorrect the entire word is counted as an incorrect spelling.
- Titles and endings: Counted in the words spelled correctly.
- Capitalization: Proper nouns must be capitalized unless the name is also a common noun. Capitalization of the first word in the sentence is not a requirement for the word to be spelled correctly. Words are counted as spelled correctly even if they are capitalized incorrectly within the sentence.
- Reversed letters: Words containing letter reversals are not counted as errors unless the reversal causes the word to be spelled incorrectly. This typically applies with reversals of the following letters: *p, q, g, d, b, n, u*.
- Contractions: In order for a contraction to be counted as correct, it must have the apostrophe in the correct place unless the word can stand alone.

QUICK SCORING GUIDE FOR WRITING CBM (CWS)

Scored as Correct

- A correct writing sequence (CWS) is "two adjacent, correctly spelled words that are acceptable within the context of the [written] phrase to a native speaker of the English language." It takes into account punctuation, syntax, semantics, spelling, and capitalization. When scoring CWS, a caret (^) is used to mark each correct word sequence. A space is implied at the beginning of a sentence.
- Spelling: Words must be spelled correctly to be counted in CWS. Words that are not counted in WSC, or are circled words, are *not* counted as CWS.
- Capitalization: Capitalization at the beginning of the sentence is necessary. Proper nouns must be capitalized unless it can serve as a common noun in the given context. Incorrectly capitalized words are marked as incorrect CWS (e.g., *Pillow, Lake*).
- Punctuation: Correct punctuation must be at the end of the sentence. Commas are not typically counted unless they are used in a series. In a series, they must be used correctly to be scored. Other punctuation marks are typically not counted as CWS.
- Syntax: Words must be syntactically correct to be counted as CWS. Sentences that begin with a conjunction are considered to be syntactically correct.
- Semantics: Words must be semantically correct to be counted in CWS.
- Story titles and endings: Story titles and endings are included in the scoring of CWS and must meet scoring criteria for spelling, punctuation, capitalization, syntax, and semantics to be counted in CWS.

QUICK ADMINISTRATION GUIDE FOR MATH CBM (MIXED-MATH)

1. Place a copy of the student sheet in front of the student(s)

2. Say: *"The sheets on your desk have math problems on them. There are several types of problems on the sheet. Some are* (insert types of problems on sheet). *Look at each problem carefully before you answer it. When I say, 'Please begin,' start answering the problems. Begin with the first problem and work across the page* (point). *Then go to the next row. If you cannot answer the problem, mark an 'X' through it and go to the next one. If you finish a page, turn the page and continue working until I say 'Thank you.' Are there any questions? Please begin."*

3. Once you say, *"Please begin,"* start the countdown timer (set for 2 minutes). At the end of 2 minutes, say: *"Thank you"* and have the student(s) put their pencils down and stop working.

Adapted from Shinn (1989)

QUICK ADMINISTRATION GUIDE FOR MATH CBM (SINGLE-SKILL)

1. Place a copy of the student sheet in front of the student(s)

2. Say: *"The sheets on your desk have* [addition, subtraction, multiplication, division, fractions, ratios, decimals, etc.] *problems on them. Look at each problem carefully before you answer it. When I say, 'Please begin,' start answering the problems. Begin with the first problem and work across the page* (point). *Then go to the next row. If you cannot answer the problem, mark an 'X' through it and go to the next one. If you finish a page, turn the page and continue working until I say 'Thank you.' Are there any questions? Please begin."*

3. Once you say, *"Please begin,"* start the countdown timer (set for 2 minutes). At the end of 2 minutes, say: *"Thank you"* and have the student(s) put their pencils down and stop working.

Adapted from Shinn (1989)

QUICK SCORING GUIDE FOR MATH CBM

Scored as Correct

- If the student has the correct answer, she is given credit for the longest method used to solve the problem *even if all the work is not shown*.
- If a problem has been crossed out or started, but not completed, the student still receives credit for any correct digits. Correct work is correct work, even if the student did not finish the problem.
- Reversed or rotated digits are scored as correct with the exception of 6's and 9's. With 6's and 9's, it is not possible to tell which one the student meant to write. No other digits can become others through rotation or reversal.
- In multiplication problems, any symbol used as a place holder is counted as a correct digit as long as it is holding a place that needs to be held. The student can use a 0, X, ☺, a blank space, or whatever else as long as it is used to hold that place.
- Parts of the answer above the line, such as carries or borrows, are not counted as correct digits. These are part of the work of the solution—not the solution itself—thus, their correctness is shown in the answer below the line.
- In division, a basic fact is when both the divisor and the quotient are 9 or less. The total CD is always 1. Also, remainders of 0 are not counted as correct digits nor are placeholders.

SURVEY-LEVEL ASSESSMENT FOR MATH

Student: _____   **Grade:** _____   **Date:** _____

Examiner: _____

Directions: Starting with the students' grade-level math sheets, have the student work on three math sheets for 2 minutes each. Count the number of digits correct for each, record the median (Mdn) digits correct score, and compare to the performance criteria. For mixed-math sheets, administer grade-level sheets and then skill-specific (math fact) sheets in areas in which difficulty was noted; or continue testing back in grade levels until the student is successfully able to meet the expected performance criteria (see below).

For each math probe assessed, use the table below to record the following

MIXED MATH						MATH FACTS					
MATH LEVEL	CORRECT DIGITS				RANGE (see below)	FACT	CORRECT DIGITS				RANGE (see below)
	#1	#2	#3	Mdn			#1	#2	#3	Mdn	
						+					
						−					
						×					
						÷					

CRITERIA FOR DETERMINING STUDENT'S INSTRUCTIONAL LEVEL

INSTRUCTIONAL LEVEL	CORRECT DIGITS (FRUSTRATIONAL RANGE)	CORRECT DIGITS (INSTRUCTIONAL RANGE)	CORRECT DIGITS (MASTERY RANGE)
1–3	0–13	14–31	32+
4+	0–23	24–49	50+

STUDENT'S PERFORMANCE GRAPH

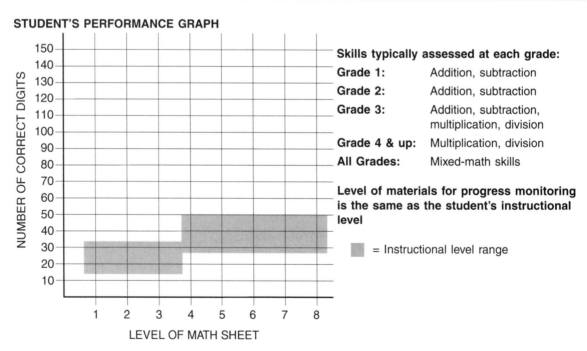

Skills typically assessed at each grade:

Grade 1: Addition, subtraction

Grade 2: Addition, subtraction

Grade 3: Addition, subtraction, multiplication, division

Grade 4 & up: Multiplication, division

All Grades: Mixed-math skills

Level of materials for progress monitoring is the same as the student's instructional level

▨ = Instructional level range

GRAPH FOR PROGRESS-MONITORING DATA

Student: _____   Teacher: _____   Grade: _____   Level: _____

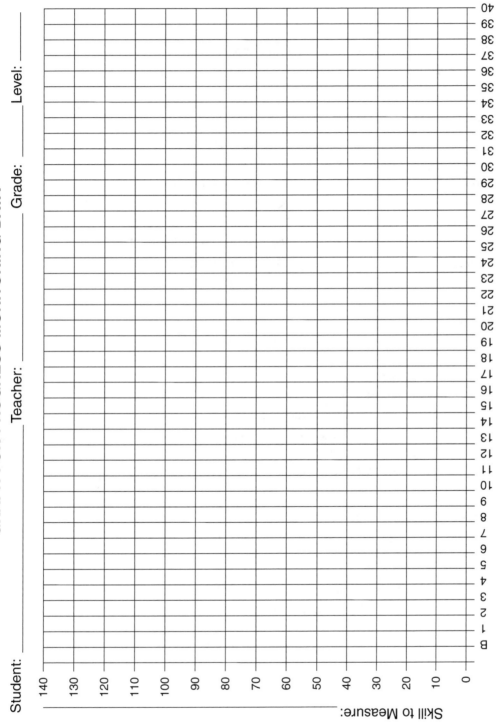

Skill to Measure: _____

Weeks

CHECKLIST FOR USING CBM BEFORE, DURING, AND AFTER INITIAL IMPLEMENTATION

BEFORE

Step 1: Who will be using CBM? (Check all that apply.)

____ Classroom(s) ____ Grade(s) ____ School(s) ____ District

Step 2: Which CBM skills will be implemented? (Check all that apply)

Early Reading	____ LSF (letter sounds)
	____ WIF (word identification)
	____ DIBELS
Reading	____ ORF (oral reading fluency)
	____ Maze
Spelling	____ CLS (correct letter sequences)
	____ WSC (words spelled correctly)
Writing	____ TWW (total words written)
	____ WSC (words spelled correctly)
	____ CWS (correct word sequences)
Math	____ Early Numeracy
	____ Computation
	____ Concepts and Applications

Step 3: What materials will we use?

____ Commercial product with graphing program

____ Purchase premade material (i.e., passages, lists, sheets, story starters) and make your own graphing program

____ Purchase premade materials (i.e., passages, lists, sheets, story starters) and graph on paper

Step 4: When will implementation start?

____ Fall ____ Winter ____ Spring

Step 5: Who will train the staff?

____ Hire a professional trainer to train the staff

____ Have a couple of staff members receive professional training and then train the rest of the staff

____ Train yourselves by using published materials and practicing together as a group

(continued)

DURING

Step 6:   Who will manage the materials?

_____ Teacher (general education, Title I, ESL, special education)

_____ Administrator (principal, vice principal)

_____ Support Staff (speech therapist, reading specialist, school psychologist)

_____ Assistants (administrative assistants, parent volunteers)

Step 7:   Who will collect the data?

_____ Individual teachers

_____ Teams (e.g., general and special education teachers, educational assistants, principals, school psychologists, reading specialists, speech therapists)

Step 8:   Where will the data be collected?

_____ In the classroom

_____ Central location (library, cafeteria, multipurpose room)

AFTER

Step 9:   Who will manage the data once they are collected?

_____ Each teacher is responsible for entering and graphing students' data

_____ One person for each grade or school is responsible for entering and graphing the data

_____ A team of people at the district is responsible for entering and graphing the data

Step 10:   How will the data be shared?

_____ Each teacher is responsible for looking at his or her own data

_____ At the grade level, all of the teachers look at all of the students together

_____ At the school level, a team is responsible for looking at all of the students

GENERAL FIDELITY CHECKLIST FOR CONDUCTING CBM

BEFORE

Yes No

☐ ☐ 1. Has the correct student material and teacher/examiner material.

☐ ☐ 2. Has a pen or pencil to mark teacher/examiner sheet.

☐ ☐ 3. Has a countdown timer that shows seconds or a stopwatch.

☐ ☐ 4. Has a clipboard and holds it so the student cannot see the teacher/examiner's materials.

DURING

Yes No

☐ ☐ 5. Reads the standardized directions verbatim.

☐ ☐ 6. Starts the stopwatch according to the directions.

☐ ☐ 7. Follows the procedure for time allowed on each item.

☐ ☐ 8. Marks the student's errors on the teacher/examiner sheet.

☐ ☐ 9. Does not correct the student when he or she makes an error (except when allowed in the example material only).

☐ ☐ 10. Follows the discontinuation rule.

☐ ☐ 11. Administers the task for the correct amount of time.

☐ ☐ 12. Stops the student at the end of the time and marks where the student stops.

AFTER

Yes No

☐ ☐ 13. Adds up the number of errors correctly.

☐ ☐ 14. Determines the total number of items attempted.

☐ ☐ 15. Scores the task by subtracting the errors from the total attempted.

☐ ☐ 16. Prorates the score if the student finishes the task before the time is up.

References

AIMSweb. (2003, April 1). *AIMSweb training workbook: Administration and scoring of early literacy measures for use with AIMSweb.* Retrieved from http://aimsweb.edformation.com/downloads/AdminandScoringEarlyLiteracy04012003.pdf

AIMSweb. (2006). *Oral reading fluency norms* [Data file]. Available at http://www.aimsweb.com

Burns, M. K., VanDerHeyden, A. M., & Jiban, C. (2006). Assessing the instructional level for mathematics: A comparison of methods. *School Psychology Review, 35,* 401–418.

Conte, K. L., & Hintze, J. M. (2000). The effects of performance feedback and goal setting on oral reading fluency within curriculum-based measurement. *Diagnostique, 25,* 85–98.

Deno, S. L. (1985). Curriculum-based measurement: The emerging alternative. *Exceptional Children, 52,* 219–232.

Deno, S. L., Fuchs, L. S., Marston, D., & Shin, J. (2001). Using curriculum-based measurement to establish growth standards for students with learning disabilities. *School Psychology Review, 30,* 507–524.

Deno, S. L., Marston, D., & Mirkin, P. K. (1982). Valid measurement procedures for continuous evaluation of written expression. *Exceptional Children, 48,* 368–371.

Deno, S. L., & Mirkin, P. K. (1977). *Data-based program modification: A manual.* Reston, VA: Council for Exceptional Children.

Deno, S. L., Mirkin, P. K., Lowry, L., & Kuehnle, K. (1980). *Relationships among simple measures of spelling and performance on standardized tests* (Research Report No. 21). Minneapolis: University of Minnesota, Institute for Research on Learning Disabilities.

DIBELS. (2006). *Benchmark goals* [Data file]. Available at http://dibels.uoregon.edu/

Edcheckup. (2005). *Administering the oral reading CBM assessment* [section 2]. Minneapolis, MN: Author.

Espin, C. A., Scierka, B. J., Skare, S., & Halverson, N. (1999). Criterion-related validity of curriculum-based measures in writing for secondary school students. *Reading and Writing Quarterly: Overcoming Learning Difficulties, 15,* 5–27.

Espin, C. A., Shin, J., Deno, S. L., Skare, S., Robinson, S., & Benner, B. (2000). Identifying indicators of written expression proficiency for middle school students. *Journal of Special Education, 34,* 140–153.

Fewster, S., & Macmillan, P. D. (2002). School-based evidence for the validity of curriculum-based measurement of reading and writing. *Remedial and Special Education, 23,* 149–156.

Fuchs, L. S., Butterworth, J. R., & Fuchs, D. (1989). Effects of ongoing curriculum-based measurement on student awareness of goals and progress. *Education and Treatment of Children, 12,* 63–72.

Fuchs, L. S., & Fuchs, D. (1991). Curriculum-based measurements: Current applications and future directions. *Preventing School Failure, 35*(3), 6–11.

Fuchs, L. S., & Fuchs, D. (2004). *Using CBM for progress monitoring.* Retrieved from http://www.studentprogress.org

Fuchs, L. S., Fuchs, D., & Hamlett, C. L. (1988). *Computer applications to curriculum-based measurement: Effects of teacher feedback systems.* Unpublished manuscript, Peabody College, Vanderbilt University, Nashville, TN.

Fuchs, L. S., Fuchs, D., & Hamlett, C. L. (1989). Computers and curriculum-based measurement: Effect of teacher feedback systems. *School Psychology Review, 18,* 112–125.

Fuchs, L. S., Fuchs, D., Hamlett, C. L., & Allinder, R. M. (1991). The contribution of skills analysis within curriculum-based measurement in spelling. *Exceptional Children, 5,* 443–452.

Fuchs, L. S., Fuchs, D., Hamlett, C. L., Walz, L., & Germann, G. (1993). Formative evaluation of academic progress: How much growth can we expect? *School Psychology Review, 22,* 27–49.

Fuchs, L. S., Fuchs, D., Hamlett, C. L., & Whinnery, K. (1991). Effects of goal line feedback on level, slope, and stability of performance within curriculum-based measurement. *Learning Disabilities Research and Practice, 6*(2), 66–74.

Gansle, K. A., Noell, G. H., VanDerHeyden, A. M., Naquin, G. M., & Slider, N. J. (2002). Moving beyond total words written: The reliability, criterion validity, and time cost of alternate measures for curriculum-based measurement in writing. *School Psychology Review, 31,* 477–497.

Gansle, K. A., Noell, G. H., VanDerHeyden, A. M., Slider, N. J., Hoffpauir, L. D., Whitmarsh, E. L., et al. (2004). An examination of the criterion validity and sensitivity to brief intervention of alternate curriculum-based measures of writing skill. *Psychology in the Schools, 41,* 291–300.

Good, R. H., III, & Jefferson, G. (1998). Contemporary perspectives on curriculum-based measurement validity. In M. R. Shinn (Ed.), *Advanced applications of curriculum-based measurement* (pp. 61–88). New York: Guilford Press.

Good, R. H., Gruba, J., & Kaminski, R. A. (2002). Best practices in using dynamic indicators of basic early literacy skills (DIBELS) in an outcomes-driven model. In A. Thomas & J. Grimes (Eds.), *Best practices in school psychology IV* (pp. 679–700). Bethesda, MD: National Association of School Psychologists.

Hasbrouck, J., & Tindal, G. A. (2006). Oral reading fluency norms: A valuable assessment tool for reading teachers. *The Reading Teacher, 59,* 636–644.

Hintze, J. M., Shapiro, E. S., Conte, K. L., & Basile, I. M. (1997). Oral reading fluency and authentic reading material: Criterion validity of the technical features of CBM survey-level assessment. *School Psychology Review, 26,* 535–553.

Howell, K. W., Hosp, J. L., Hosp, M. K., & Macconell, K. (in press). *Curriculum-based evaluation: Linking assessment and instruction.* New York: Sage.

Hutton, J. B., Dubes, R., & Muir, S. (1992). Estimating trend progress in monitoring data: A comparison of simple line-fitting methods. *School Psychology Review, 21,* 300–312.

Jenkins, J. R., Fuchs, L. S., van den Broek, P., Espin, C. A., & Deno, S. L. (2003). Sources of individual differences in reading comprehension and reading fluency. *Journal of Educational Psychology, 95,* 719–729.

Jewell, J., & Malecki, C. K. (2003). The utility of written language indices: An investigation production dependent, production independent, and accurate production scores. *School Psychology Review, 34,* 27–44.

Loeffer, K. A. (2005). No more Friday spelling test? *Teaching Exceptional Children, 37*(4), 24–27.

Madelaine, A., & Wheldall, K. (1998). Towards a curriculum-based passage reading test for monitoring the performance of low-progress readers using standardized passages: A validity study. *Educational Psychology, 18,* 471–478.

Malecki, C. K., & Jewell, J. (2003). Developmental, gender, and practical considerations in scoring curriculum-based writing probes. *Psychology in the Schools, 40,* 379–390.

Marston, D. B. (1982). The technical adequacy of direct, repeated measurement of academic skills in low achieving elementary students. (Doctoral dissertation, University of Minnesota, 1982). *Dissertation Abstracts International, 43,* AAT 8301966.

Marston, D. B. (1983). *A comparison of standardized achievement tests and direct measurement techniques in measuring pupil progress* (Research Report No. 50). Minneapolis: University of Minnesota, Institute for Research on Learning Disabilities.

Marston, D. B. (1989). A curriculum-based measurement approach to assessing academic performance: What it is and why do it. In M. R. Shinn (Ed.), *Curriculum-based measurement: Assessing special children* (pp. 18–78). New York: Guilford Press.

Marston, D. B., Mirkin, P., & Deno, S. (1984). Curriculum-based measurement: An alternative to traditional screening, referral, and identification. *The Journal of Special Education, 18*, 109–117.

National Institute Child Health & Human Development. (2000, April). *Report of the National Reading Panel: Teaching Children to Read.* Washington, DC: Author.

Powell-Smith, K. A., & Shinn, M. R. (2004). *Administration and scoring of written expression curriculum-based measurement for use in general outcome measurement.* Eden Prairie, MN. Edformation.

Shapiro, E. S. (2004). *Academic skills problems: Direct assessment and intervention* (3rd ed.). New York: Guilford Press.

Shinn, M. R. (1981). A comparison of psychometric and functional differences between students labeled learning disabled and low achieving. (Doctoral dissertation, University of Minnesota, 1981). *Dissertation Abstracts International, 42*, AAT 8275871.

Shinn, M. R. (1989). *Curriculum-based measurement: Assessing special children.* New York: Guilford Press.

Shinn, M. R., & Shinn, M. M. (2002a). *AIMSweb training workbook: Administration and scoring of early literacy measures for use with AIMSweb.* Eden Prairie, MN: Edformation.

Shinn, M. R., & Shinn, M. M. (2002b). *AIMSweb training workbook: Administration and scoring of reading maze for use in general outcome measurement.* Eden Prairie, MN: Edformation.

Shinn, M. R., Ysseldyke, J. E., Deno, S. L., & Tindal, G. A. (1986). A comparison of differences between students labeled learning disabled and low achieving on measures of classroom performance. *Journal of Learning Disabilities, 19*, 545–552.

Skiba, R., Magnusson, D., Marston, D. B., & Erickson, K. (1986). *The assessment of mathematics performance in special education: Achievement tests, proficiency tests, or formative evaluation?* Minneapolis: Special Services, Minneapolis Public Schools.

Snow, C. E., Burns, M. S., & Griffin, P. (Eds.). (1998). *Preventing reading difficulties in young children.* Washington, DC: National Academy Press.

Thurber, R. S., Shinn, M. R., & Smolkowski, K. (2002). What is measured in mathematics tests?: Construct validity of curriculum-based mathematics measures. *School Psychology Review, 31*, 498–513.

Tindal, G., Germann, G., & Deno, S. L. (1983). *Descriptive research on the pine county norms: A compilation of findings* (Research Report No. 132). Minneapolis: University of Minnesota Institute for Research on Learning Disabilities.

Tindal, G., Marston, D. B., & Deno, S. L. (1983). *The reliability of direct and repeated measurement* (Research Report No. 109). Minneapolis: University of Minnesota Institute for Research on Learning Disabilities.

Tindal, G., & Parker, R. (1989). Assessment of written expression for students in compensatory and special education programs. *Journal of Special Education, 23*, 169–183.

Tindal, G., & Parker, R. (1991). Identifying measures for evaluating written expression. *Learning Disabilities: Research and Practice, 6*, 211–218.

Videen, J., Deno, S, & Marston, D. B. (1982). *Correct word sequences: A valid indicator of written expression* (Rep. No. 84). Minneapolis, MN.

Watkinson, J. T., & Lee, S. W. (1992). Curriculum-based measures of written expression for learning-disabled and non-disabled students. *Psychology in the Schools, 29*, 184–191.

Weiner, J. (1986). Alternatives in the assessment of the learning disabled adolescent: A learning strategies approach. *Learning Disabilities Focus, 1*, 97–107.

Index

Abbreviations, scoring CBMs and, 39, 89, 90, 146, 154
Academic failure, risk of, 45, 55
Administration of CBM measures
    frequency of CBMs, 44–46, 67
    ORF and Maze CBMs, 145
    overview, 16–17
    planning the use of CBMs and, 138, 140
    quick guides and forms for, 145–146, 147–148, 162
    time needed for CBMs, 46, 68
Advantages of CBM, 8–9
AIMSweb, 15, 33, 99, 129
Alignment, principle of, 3–4, 7, 8–9, 18, 22
Alternate variables, 6
Articulation problems, 38, 62, 66, 146, 151
    letter sound fluency (LSF) CBM and, 62
Assessment, 18

B

Behavior data, 4, 5, 22
Benchmarks
    frequency of administration, 45, 93
    LSF and WIF CBMs, 67
    math CBM, 108, 116
    overview, 20, 25–26, 26–27
    planning the use of CBMs and, 139
    reading CBMs and, 48, 48t
    setting and graphing goals and, 120–123
    spelling CBM and, 78
    writing CBM, 93–94

C

Capitalization, scoring CBMs and, 90–91, 153, 154, 155
Charting CBM data
    computerized systems for, 127–130
    frequency of, 123–124
    overview, 118, 118–120, 119f, 120f, 126, 130–131
    planning the use of CBMs and, 134, 137
Contractions, scoring writing CBM and, 91, 154
Counting skills, 115
Criterion-referenced measures, 4, 7–8, 22–24, 23, 25–26
Curriculum, 3, 5–6, 17–18, 98, 130
Curriculum-based evaluation (CBE), 17

D

Data-based decision making, 9–10
Data-Based Program Modification (DBPM), 3, 9
Data from CBMs. *See also* Charting CBM data; Graphing CBM data
    computerized systems for graphing and charting, 127–130
    decision making and, 124–125, 125f
    form for, 159
    frequency of collection, 123–124
    overview, 118, 130–131
    planning the use of CBMs and, 134, 136–138
    response to intervention model and, 126–127
Data gathering, decision making and, 20, 22

Decision-making
  data from CBMs and, 9, 18, 124–125, 125*f*
  overview, 19, 20–22, 26–27
  progress-monitoring and, 27–29
  relating RTI to CBM and, 9–10
  response to intervention model and, 126–127
Designing CBMs, curriculum and, 17–18
Diagnostic decisions
  administration of CBM and, 17
  math CBM, 110, 112–113, 113*f*
  overview, 9, 21
  progress-monitoring and, 29
Dialect, scoring CBMs and, 38, 62, 66, 146, 151
Directions for CBMs
  letter sound fluency (LSF) CBM, 59–60
  math CBM, 104, 156
  for Maze CBM, 42–44, 42*f*
  for ORF CBM, 35–39, 35*f*, 36*f*
  quick guides and forms for, 145–146, 147–148,
    150, 151, 154
  spelling CBM and, 75–76, 152
  word identification fluency (WIF) CBM, 64–
    65, 64*f*, 65*f*
  writing CBM, 88–92, 89*f*
Dual discrepancy method, 127
Dynamic Indicators of Basic Early Literacy Skills
    (DIBELS)
  benchmarks for ORF CBM, 48*t*
  compared to CBM, 70
  computerized systems for graphing and
    charting CBM data, 128
  early reading skills and, 31–32, 55–56
  overview, 14–15, 33, 56–57
  planning the use of, 133

E

Early numeracy skills, 113–115, 114*f*
Early reading CBM. *See also* Letter sound
    fluency (LSF) CBM; Reading CBM; Word
    identification fluency (WIF) CBM
  Dynamic Indicators of Basic Early Literacy
    Skills (DIBELS), 56–57
  FAQs regarding, 70
  frequency of administration, 67
  growth rates and norms for, 68, 68*t*, 69*t*
  letter sound fluency (LSF) CBM, 57–63, 59*f*,
    60*f*, 61*f*
  planning the use of, 133
  reasons to conduct, 55–56
  time needed for, 68

  using data from for IEP goals and objectives,
    69–70
  word identification fluency (WIF) CBM, 63–
    67, 64*f*, 65*f*
Early reading skills, 31. *See also* Early reading
    CBM; Reading skills
Edcheckup, 15, 34, 128–129
Educational decision-making. *See* Decision-
    making
Efficiency of CBM, 5, 8–9
Errors on teacher/examiner copy, 112
Estimation, 115
Excel, 130

F

FileMaker Pro, 130
Formative evaluation, 9
Frequency of CBM administration, 44–46, 67, 78,
    93, 108

G

General outcome measures, 9, 10–11, 15*t*, 28, 29
Goals
  LSF and WIF CBMs and, 69
  math CBM and, 111–112
  ORF and Maze CBMs and, 51–52
  planning the use of CBMs and, 139–140
  setting and graphing, 120–123
  spelling CBM and, 80
  writing CBM and, 94
Graphing CBM data
  computerized systems for, 127–130
  form for, 159
  frequency of, 123–124
  goals and, 123
  overview, 118, 126, 130–131
  planning the use of CBMs and, 134, 137
Group administration of CBM, 16

H

Handwriting, 96
Hesitations, scoring CBMs and, 38, 62, 66, 146,
    150, 151
History of CBM, 3
Hyphenated words, scoring CBMs and, 39, 89,
    90, 146, 153, 154

I

IEP goals and objectives
  LSF and WIF CBMs and, 69–70
  math CBM and, 111–112
  ORF and Maze CBMs and, 51–52
  planning the use of CBMs and, 139–140
  spelling CBM and, 80
  writing CBM and, 94
Individual differences among students, 25
Inferences. *See* Low-inference measures
Initial sound fluency (ISF), 56
Insertions, scoring CBMs and, 38, 146, 153
Instruction
  CBM and, 10, 17–18, 124–125, 125*f*
  criterion-referenced measures and, 7
  response to intervention model and, 126–127
  skills-based measures and, 12
Instructional decisions, 22
Instructional grouping, 53, 70, 82, 116
Internet resources, 30, 98, 99–100, 128–129
Interpretations of CBM scores, 18
Intervention Central, 34, 129
Interventions, 10
Intraindividual framework, 122–123

L

Learning disabilities, 84, 127. *See also* IEP goals
    and objectives
Letter naming fluency (LNF), 57
Letter–sound fluency (LSF) CBM. *See also* Early
    reading CBM
  FAQs regarding, 70
  frequency of administration, 67
  growth rates and norms for, 68, 68*t*, 69*t*
  overview, 57–63, 59*f*, 60*f*, 61*f*
  planning the use of, 133
  quick guides and forms for, 150
  time needed for, 68
  using data from for IEP goals and objectives,
    69–70
Low-inference measures, 4, 6–7

M

Mastery measures
  comparing to other forms of measurement, 11, 15*t*
  overview, 9, 12–14, 13*f*, 14*f*
  progress-monitoring and, 29

Materials, CBM
  Internet resources, 30
  letter sound fluency (LSF) CBM, 57–59
  math CBM, 98–103, 101*f*, 102*f*, 103*f*
  overview, 18
  planning the use of CBMs and, 133, 134, 135–
    136, 139, 160, 160–161
  spelling CBM and, 72–74, 74*f*, 75*f*
  word identification fluency (WIF) CBM, 63–64
  writing CBM and, 85, 86*f*, 87, 87*f*
Math CBM
  directions and scoring procedures for, 104–
    107, 105*f*
  FAQs regarding, 116
  frequency of administration, 108
  growth rates and norms for, 109–110, 109*t*,
    110*t*, 111*t*
  materials needed for, 98–103, 101*f*, 102*f*, 103*f*
  quick guides and forms for, 156–158
  reasons to conduct, 97
  reliability and validity studies regarding, 142
  special considerations that apply to, 112–115,
    113*f*, 114*f*
  survey-level assessment with, 110
  time needed for, 108
  using data from for IEP goals and objectives,
    111–112
Math computation, 11–12
Maze CBM
  directions and scoring procedures for, 42–44,
    42*f*
  frequency of administration, 44–46
  growth rates and norms for, 46–48, 47*t*, 48*t*, 50*t*
  materials needed for, 40
  overview, 32, 40, 41*f*, 42–44, 42*f*, 53–54
  planning the use of, 133
  quick guides and forms for, 147–148
  reading passages for, 40, 41*f*
  resources for, 33–34
  time needed for, 46
  using data from for IEP goals and objectives,
    51–52
Minneapolis Public Schools, 99
Monitoring Basic Skills Progress (PRO-ED), 34,
    99, 129
Multilevel Academic Skills Inventory (MASI), 29

N

Nonsense word fluency (NWF), 57
Norm-referenced tests (NRTs), 22–24

Norm sampling, 25
Norms
    establishing performance standards and, 25
    for LSF and WIF CBMs, 68, 68f, 69f
    math CBM and, 109–110, 109t, 110t, 111t
    norm-referenced tests and, 22
    ORF and Maze CBMs and, 46–48, 47t, 48,
        48t, 49t–50t
    overview, 22–23
    setting and graphing goals and, 121–122
    spelling CBM and, 79–80, 81t
    writing CBM, 93–94, 95t
Numerals, 39, 146

O

Objectives
    LSF and WIF CBMs and, 69–70
    math CBM and, 111–112
    ORF and Maze CBMs and, 51–52
    planning the use of CBMs and, 139–140
    spelling CBM and, 80
    writing CBM and, 94
Omissions, scoring CBMs and, 38, 62, 66, 146,
    150, 151
Oral reading fluency, 11, 32. See also Oral
        reading fluency CBM; Reading skills
Oral reading fluency CBM. See also Reading
        CBM
    directions and scoring procedures for, 35–39,
        35f, 36f
    frequency of administration, 44–46
    growth rates and norms for, 46–48, 47t, 48t, 49t
    materials needed for, 32–35
    overview, 32–39, 53–54
    planning the use of, 133
    quick guides and forms for, 145–146, 149
    reading passages for, 33–35
    resources for, 33–34
    survey-level assessment with, 51
    time needed for, 46
    using data from for IEP goals and objectives,
        51–52
Outcome decisions, 9, 21

P

Performance criteria, 22, 25–26, 26–27, 45, 110,
    120–123
Phoneme segmentation fluency (PSF), 56

Planning, CBM use and, 132–138, 138–139, 139–
    140, 160–162
Predictive validity model, 25
Preparations involved in administering CBM,
    16
Problem-solving process, 6, 9–10, 19
Productive thinking, 20
Professional training and development, 53, 70,
    130–135, 160
Proficiency levels, 48, 48t, 68. See also
    Benchmarks
Program-specific measurements, 17–18
Progress monitoring with CBM
    charting and graphing CBM data and, 131
    criterion-referenced measures and, 8
    decision-making from CBM data and, 9, 21,
        26–27
    form for, 159
    frequency of administration, 45, 93
    LSF and WIF CBMs and, 67
    math CBM and, 98, 108
    norms and, 121–122
    ORF and Maze CBMs and, 45, 46–48, 47t,
        48t, 49t–50t
    overview, 4–5, 8–9, 27–29, 139
    skills-based measures and, 12
    spelling CBM and, 78
Project AIM, 34
Pronunciation, scoring CBMs and, 37, 38, 60–61,
    66, 146, 150, 151
Punctuation, 92, 155

R

Reading CBM. See also Early reading CBM;
        Maze CBM; Oral reading fluency CBM
    FAQs regarding, 53–54
    frequency of administration, 44–46
    planning the use of, 133
    reasons to conduct, 31–32, 32t
    reliability and validity studies regarding, 141,
        142
    using data from for IEP goals and objectives,
        51–52
Reading First legislation, 20–22
Reading passages for CBM, 33–35, 40, 41f
Reading skills, 31–32. See also Early reading
        skills
Reliability of measures, 22, 24–25, 142
Repeated measurement, 4
Repetitions, scoring CBMs and, 38, 146, 153

Research Institute on Progress Monitoring, 99
Resources
    CBM materials, 18
    computerized systems for graphing and
        charting CBM data, 127–130
    early reading CBMs and, 71
    Internet resources, 30
    math CBM, 99–100
    reading CBMs and, 33–34, 54, 58
    spelling lists, 73
    story starters, 85
Response to intervention (RTI) model, 9–10, 30,
    126–127
Reversals, scoring CBMs and, 38–39, 62, 66–67,
    91, 146, 150, 151, 154, 157

S

Scheduling, 139
Scoring of CBMs, 46
Scoring rules
    decision making and, 22
    letter sound fluency (LSF) CBM, 59–63, 59f,
        60f, 61f
    math CBM, 104–107, 105f, 157
    for Maze CBM, 42–44, 42f
    for ORF CBM, 35–39, 35f, 36f, 146
    overview, 18
    quick guides and forms for, 146, 150, 151,
        154–155
    reading CBMs and, 53
    scoring spelling CBMs and, 153
    word identification fluency (WIF) CBM, 64–
        67
    writing CBM, 88–92, 89f
Screening decisions
    frequency of CBM administration, 45, 93
    LSF and WIF CBMs, 67
    math CBM and, 98, 108
    overview, 9, 20
    planning the use of CBMs and, 139
    spelling CBM and, 78
    using CBM for, 26–27
Self-corrections, scoring CBMs and, 38, 61,
    66, 146, 150, 151
Semantics, scoring writing CBM and, 92,
    155
Skills-based measures, 9, 11–12, 15t, 28, 29
Skills, mastery measures and, 13
Special education, 16, 17, 127, 139–140
Specific-level assessment, 9

Spelling CBM
    directions and scoring procedures for, 75–78
    FAQs regarding, 80, 82
    frequency of administration, 78
    growth rates and norms for, 79–80, 81t
    materials needed for, 72–74, 74f, 75f
    planning the use of, 133
    quick guides and forms for, 152–153
    reasons to conduct, 72
    reliability and validity studies regarding, 141,
        142
    time needed for, 78–79
    using data from for IEP goals and objectives,
        80
Spelling lists, 73–74, 74f, 75f
Spelling skills, scoring writing CBM and, 90–91,
    155
Standardized measures, 22, 24
Standards
    establishing, 25–26
    norms and criterion and, 23
    ORF and Maze CBMs and, 46–48, 47t, 48t
    setting and graphing goals and, 120–123
Story starters for writing CBMs, 85, 86f, 87,
    87f
Struggling students, 45. See also IEP goals and
    objectives
Survey-level assessment
    form for, 149
    math CBM and, 98, 108, 110, 158
    with ORF CBM, 45–46, 51
    overview, 9
Syntax, scoring writing CBM and, 92, 155
Systems based interventions, 6

T

Technical adequacy of CBM, 4
Time involved in administering CBMs, 46,
    68, 78–79, 93, 108
Tool skills, mastery measures and, 13
Training in using CBMs, 53, 70, 134–135,
    160
Types of CBM, 9, 10–14, 13f, 14f, 15t

V

Validity of measures, 22, 24–25, 141–142
Vanderbilt University, 34, 99–100
Variability on measures, 23–24

W

Word identification fluency (WIF) CBM. *See also* Early reading CBM
   FAQs regarding, 70
   frequency of administration, 67
   growth rates and norms for, 68, 68*t*, 69*t*
   overview, 63–67, 64*f*, 65*f*
   planning the use of, 133
   quick guides and forms for, 151
   time needed for, 68
   using data for IEP goals and objectives, 69–70
Word substitutions, 66, 151
Writing CBM
   directions and scoring procedures for, 88–92, 89*f*
   FAQs regarding, 94, 96
   frequency of administration, 93
   growth rates and norms for, 93–94, 95*t*
   planning the use of, 133
   quick guides and forms for, 154–155
   reasons to conduct, 84
   reliability studies regarding, 142
   time needed for, 93
   using data from for IEP goals and objectives, 94
   validity studies regarding, 141

Y

Yearly Progress Pro, 34, 99–100, 129